"Cancer and Me"

"Cancer; the Body and Minds Silent Destroyer"

David Keough

**A Donation of £1 from each book sale will go directly to
Cancer Research**

Note to self

"Maintain a Positive Mental Attitude"

"When I began my journey of treatment for

Cancer;

I was focused to be where I am today.

If I give up, I will end up back where I started.

*With perseverance and courage I will overcome
this disease"*

Dedication

There are so many people who this book is dedicated to; the outstanding service, care and professionalism of the multi-disciplinary medical teams. Without them, I would not be here today; words do not describe the lengths they go to, making sure you have the best care and treatment they can give you, day and night.

To my wife Fatima who has walked every step of the way with me, shared the highs and lows, never faltering and always believing we would get through this together. Wesley, Simone and Claire, our children, always on hand to help; and to the close friends and family who showed their continued support and care, not just for me, for all of us as a family.

To John and the ladies in the office; Julie, Anita and Marje for understanding and careful scheduling of my work appointments and ensuring I am working within the legal guidelines for chemotherapy treatment, my capabilities and not over stretching it; it's a difficult task the best of times, without me putting a spanner in the works.

Without any single one of you, the journey would have been a lot more painful and a great deal harder to make; thank you all

Foreword

Cancer is never far away from the news; it now affects every 1 in 2 people, a statistic that I still find quite staggering. Despite all the research and development into finding a cure, were great strides have been made; cancer still manages to raise its ugly head, continually destroying lives.

I have heard so many stories about cancer and the affects it has on their lives, and the lives of their loved ones. The success stories, the sad stories and stories from people still on their journey.

With all the information being fired at you, it can become quite overwhelming and confusing, sometimes not knowing which way to turn or what question to ask. I thought I would give a day by day account of my journey, no watering down or exaggeration, just a very honest and frank account.

I believe it helped me deal with my cancer, by putting my thoughts, feelings and actions down on paper, to stop them whirling around my head, possibly creating problems that don't exist by over thinking, listening too much to the voices of doom in my head. With all this confusion and uncertainty, it's like having a runaway freight train hurtling through your mind with no station in sight to bring it to a halt

I hope it will help you and your family understand your journey; you are not alone and you are far more important to other people, than to allow cancer to ruin yours and their lives.

Every person will have a different experience when they have cancer, it is not one size fits all; our type of cancer will be different, our chemotherapy will be different, our side effects will be different; everything around cancer is individualised. The one thing we all have in common, we all have a battle on our hands wishing for the same outcome of being cured; it is just our approaches, our journey and mind-sets that will be different.

 The journey is going to be tough, very tough; there are no easy fixes for cancer; it does not discriminate against age, culture or gender. It has one sole purpose, to take up residency in our bodies and to unleash havoc on us, playing games with our emotions, trying to destroy our will to live, wanting us to give up at every opportunity and to ultimately take our life. Cancer lays down the gauntlet to the medical teams; a challenge they are always up for and always want to conquer.

My journey will not be a sprint to the finish line, rather more like a marathon; with perseverance, irrespective of what cancer throws at me, I will cross that finish line. Cancer will try and fool you, having you think that it is the end of cancer once your hair starts to grow back after chemotherapy. Don't get lured into this false pretence; this disease will try again and again to raise its ugly face. If you are somewhere on your journey, believe in yourself and believe in the medical teams who are looking after you; they are truly amazing at their profession and as human beings, they also share our ups and downs, and never falter to be with you on your journey.

There is so much emphasis being placed on save the planet, reducing carbon emissions and reducing plastic (quite rightly so), by countries around the world, they can now see how the planet is being destroyed. If cancer is affecting every 1 in every 2 people, 50% of the world population, surely cancer should have the same importance placed on it. This is why we need to support Cancer Research, to help them one day find a permanent cure against cancer and rid us all of this disease; only then can we all breathe more easily. We as an individual cannot do a massive amount in finding a cure for cancer; however, we can all play a small collective part in doing so. By purchasing this book; £1 from every book sale will go directly to Cancer Research; that is a significant start in raising vital funds for research.

Please support Cancer Research; even if a cure is not found in my life time, I hope it is for my own children and grandchildren; they need our continued support now, to make this happen.

Sequence of Events

- August 13th Appointment with my GP-Dr B
- August 17th Endoscopy at Harrogate Hospital
- August 20th CT Scan at Harrogate Hospital
- September 4th Diagnosis Results
- September 9th Phone call from Dr B
- September 10th Appointment with the Dietician
- September 11th PET Scan at St. James Hospital Leeds
- September 17th Diagnosis Results
- September 19th CPEX at LGI (heart and lung fitness)
- September 24th first meeting with the surgeon Mr s and Oncologist Consultant Dr U St James Hospital Leeds
- October1st Sign Consent forms and decontamination wash
- October 7th Pre Assessment for Chemotherapy
- October 9th PICC Lines get inserted
- October 10th Chemotherapy Cycle One and following days.
- October 22nd Pre Assessment for Chemotherapy Cycle Two
- October 24th Chemotherapy Cycle Two and following days
- November 5th Pre Assessment for Chemotherapy Cycle Three
- November 7th Chemotherapy Cycle Three and following days
- November 19th Pre Assessment for Chemotherapy Cycle Four
- November 21st Chemotherapy Cycle Four and following days
- December 5th Chemotherapy cycles finished, visit to see Dr U the Oncologist Consultant. & CT Scan at the LGI
- November 12th Results of the chemotherapy treatment
- December 20th A&E
- January 7th Meet Mr D (Surgeon) & Pre Assessment for surgery
- January 9th Surgery
- Conclusion

August 13th Appointment with my GP-Dr B

My wife Fatima and youngest daughter made me a routine Doctors appointment at my local surgery as I was having a few concerns when trying to swallow certain foods, mainly bread. This tended to become stuck in my oesophagus; it felt like someone had put a plug in a sink and the bowl kept on filling up; the only relief was to vomit whatever was stuck, out. For my part I thought nothing of it, I had just eaten too quickly and not chewed my food enough, my own fault as I'm always dashing around at 100mph. How far I was from the truth of what was really happening inside me.

I attended the appointment as arranged; and Dr B had a very strong sense of what was causing the issue of food getting stuck in my oesophagus; after a few questions, he informed me he was going to arrange an emergency appointment at the Harrogate hospital for an endoscopy to be done.

Ok I thought and went on my way not giving it too much consideration as to what Dr B had said; we all lead busy lives and my mind was already on my drive up to Scotland, as this appointment had set me back a couple of hours of my journey.

I have to admit, I never in a million years thought it was cancer that had taken up residency in my body; I cannot tell you why I did not think it was cancer, even now; I thought a lot of fuss over nothing and a quick course of an anti-biotic will clear it up.

August 17th Endoscopy at Harrogate Hospital

After leaving my Doctors I travelled up to Scotland for work as planned; I was working up there for two days around the Glasgow and Edinburgh areas. The journey was uneventful and as always, I enjoyed the beautiful scenery the UK has to offer us. For the whole of the journey, I did not give a single thought to being at the Doctors and my main focus of attention was on the work at hand.

It was two days later whilst sitting in my Van in Cambridge Street Car Park, Just getting ready to leave Glasgow when my phone rang; it was the hospital in Harrogate. They had arranged for me to have an appointment, an endoscopy on this coming Saturday afternoon, 17th August. "Yes, I will be back for the appointment" was my reply, still not giving much thought to my situation, I just remember thinking, that was pretty quick to get an appointment.

I arrived at the Hospital in plenty of time; my wife dropped me off just in case they had to sedate me and I was unable to drive afterwards. Being a Saturday the Hospital was fairly quiet, not the normal hustles and bustles one may expect from a busy place.

I made my way to the endoscopy department and checked in; there were only two other people waiting in a clean comfortable waiting area.

The Nurse called me through and checked all my details to make sure I am who I am, and everything is up to date.

An upper endoscopy allows a medical team to look at the upper part of the gastrointestinal (GI) tract. This area is made up of the; Oesophagus, which is the muscular tube that connects the throat to the stomach, Stomach, Duodenum, which is the top of the small intestine.

From there I was taken to the endoscopy room were a spray was administered to the back of my mouth; this will numb the back of my throat to help ease the swallowing of the endoscope tube. Lying now on my side, with a mouth piece in place to stop me from closing my mouth, the tube is inserted; goodness me, do I want to gag and get this thing out? Once the tube was in, it was not too bad, just the initial swallowing of it was the hardest bit.

The Gastroenterologist and his medical team then took some biopsies from my oesophagus and had a good poke around the stomach, bowels and intestines.

Once it was finished, which took about 20 minutes, I was to have a seat in a recovery ward. There were six beds in the ward, all empty; I was the only person there apart from about five medical staff. I was sat on a chair in the middle of this recovery ward, and knew then that something was not right and that they had found something that should not have been there in my oesophagus. Observing the nurses, observing and listening to the unspoken messages, I knew then this was not going to be straight forward; this was the first time the seriousness of the situation started to dawn on me. Sitting in a very quiet recovery ward; it was the first time I have ever felt alone, helpless and not in control of the situation I found myself in at this stage, staring at the floor hearing but not listening. My thoughts and emotions where all over the place, as uncontrollable feelings, kept flooding my mind, racing away in different directions to try and make sense of what was happening here. Sitting in the middle of this ward, I imagined it as I was sitting on a stage in front of a large audience, thousands of eyes staring at me from the darkness that shrouded me, in complete silence, so quiet you could hear a pin drop, lights dimmed apart from a spotlight shining on me, with a caption, "It's you". When I think back to this moment, it felt like the darkness was my only friend, and I just wanted it to swallow me up. At this stage, nothing had been said to me; I just sensed it from the reactions of the medical staff, it is about understanding the unspoken message. However, I still believed it was very unfair to push them for answers, as they are not allowed to say and I was trying to keep everything in perspective.

The gastroenterologist popped out and said to me, he had found a suspicious growth and was not happy with what he had just seen and I was to just wait a while in the recovery ward. A nurse took some blood samples, and even then the conversation was steered away from the endoscopy that I had just had, as to avoid a slip of the tongue or inadvertently saying something that could be misinterpreted.

I have to mention, the medical team were great, very caring and very professional from start to finish.

After I had finished my assessment at the hospital, my wife then picked me up to take me home. On the journey she naturally asked me how it went; I just said "fine, they will send me the results soon" I did not wish to tell her whilst she was driving, not knowing 100% how she would react to the news, that they found something suspicious growing in my oesophagus.

When we did arrive home, I told her the news; apart from the obvious questions; she was very quiet trying to take in what I had just told her. I knew she was suffering inside, but I had to let her process the information and deal with it in her own way.

We had an important event coming up soon, our eldest daughter was getting married in Italy and we as a family and friends were going to spend a long weekend in each other's company; for me, it was imperative that this unwelcome news did not come out at all before or during the wedding. This weekend was for my daughter and future son in law and I wanted to have no distractions or side shows to spoil or dampen the excitement of the happy couple and guests who would be in attendance.

I sat down and thought this through very carefully of how I want this to play out; I must have control of this and will let the people close to me who should know on my terms. I am not a control freak; however this was my illness and I need to deal with it in my own way; nothing had been confirmed to say it was cancer; but I knew it was.

So how am I going to make sure I control this? I let my two brothers know about the situation for various reasons; they both remained very tight lipped about it; and a very close, trusted friend of mine, Steve who knows me better than anyone else. I knew I could trust all three to remain quiet and not let anything slip, even as the Italian wine flowed at the wedding.

By this stage I had accepted the news that I had cancer of the oesophagus, that was the best thing I did, accept it and remove the emotion out of the situation; I was now at peace with myself. I had to make my mind stronger than my emotions to ensure my mind-set stayed healthy and in the right place. This helped me take an approach of reality, being logical and rational in my thought process. Am I going to get angry? "No", why should I punish myself even further by getting angry and blaming myself for something I did not cause; Cancer would love that. Am I going to fight this with everything I've got? "No", how can I fight it and waste my energy on something I cannot control; neither will I breakdown and cry, blame someone or something; this is a complete waste of time, energy and will only create a mind-set of defeat, doom and gloom. "No", this is not going to be like this, I am not going to have victim mentality.

I laid down a number of ground rules with my wife once the news would become common knowledge. There are a number of reasons why I wanted to control this and requested politely for people not to phone me. That decision was not to cut myself off from people, far from it; this was to help me maintain a positive mental state and keep my mind focused on getting better.

Some of the rules I made were very simple; and it was the best decision I made; it worked for me, and would do it again if needed to.

- I did not want phone calls; I find repeating the same conversation over and over becomes tiring, monotonous and frustrating. Being constantly asked the same questions again and again, questions I do not know the answers to, can become very irritating. To me, it keeps returning me to the start, giving a feeling of never moving forward; by not moving forward, it makes the situation I find myself in far greater than it already is, and reduces the chance of overcoming it. If not careful, holding people's minds in the past can have a negative effect on the mind; this can lead to other complications, an unhealthy mind has an unhealthy effect on the body-my psychology affects my physiology. I understand that people are trying to be kind and caring; please understand the words you are using, as they all have a consequence on the person you are speaking them to, not all of those consequences are positive.

- I did not want to hear others tales of success and woes surrounding cancer; every person is different and putting everyone through the same car wash of treatment does not attain the same results. Listening to others can also create a competition of whose was more serious, whose was the toughest to get through, who stared death in the face and how much they suffered. Whilst I appreciate they have gone through very tough times, and understand the difficulties of their plight, I need a clear mind and to concentrate on the information from my medical team only. They know my situation and the best treatment for me. Unfortunately' when you become poorly, people can become an expert in your illness. Family and friends have to listen to understand what I am saying and trying to achieve, rather than just listening to reply-Please, it Is not helpful

- I made a conscious effort not to use the internet; there are far too many stories and information unsubstantiated out there. When having cancer; there is so much information given to you, it is very easy to become overwhelmed. The information from Macmillan Cancer Support and the medical teams is superb, easily explained and more than enough to inform me of my situation and the treatment process they have specifically tailored for me.

- I decided so I have a clear and uncluttered mind; if I received any treatment or news, I would send the same message to the people who I need to know; this way they keep moving forward with me; it keeps me focused on my goal and focuses their minds on the positive.

- To accept there in nothing really that I can do to get rid of the cancer, I cannot do that. The only thing I can do is to follow the advice from the medical team to the letter to fulfil my side of the deal, follow the diet information and a life style reset. The other side of the deal, which can do something about the cancer, are the medical team. They have the skill, knowledge, dedication and the will to fulfil their side; and they will do their upmost. Just listen to these people and blank out the rest, it just becomes a noisy irritant otherwise.
- To ensure that when family and friends do speak to me; please bear in mind, generally my wife is at home with me and my children. Please do not forget to ask them how they are doing; they go through this journey every step of the way. Please do not forget about them, their feelings and how they are doing. This is vitally important for me and for them; please do not let them become forgotten about at this time.

- I had to correct some family members and friends for mentioning to my wife; given with all the best intentions "she has to be strong for the family, she has to be strong for herself, she has to be strong for me" This could not be any further from the truth. My wife has to deal with it the best way she knows; if that means crying, then cry; if that means shouting, then shout and so on. Not dealing with it in Fatima's own way and telling her to be strong; does not allow her to process her feelings and emotions in a natural way, specific to her; instead it forces her to bury them. This will have a negative impact on her later on in life, those buried emotions will surface come back when least expected. Again, be very careful of the words and advice you are giving; the consequences can be devastating. It is not a competition about strong or weak, right or wrong, it is about people and not a dry technical process
- I did not broadcast it to the world; sympathy does not help anybody; sympathy only allows the person giving

the sympathy a chance to take on part of my problem. That is not healthy for them and can render them ineffective; giving sympathy causes them to sit in my problem puddle with me, sharing my problem. I need empathy at this time, a clear vision.

- I left any reading material, notes, and information out in the house, so anyone could pick them up and understand more about cancer and my treatment if they felt embarrassed to ask.

- I accepted the journey to recovery is going to be very tough; each tough day means that it is one step closer to my finish line. If I don't have a rough day; then that is a bonus.

- To maintain a positive, healthy mind, I focused on the situation I was in and the outcome I wanted; and not the situation I was in and the outcome I didn't want. Positive thinking versus negative thinking. It is about facing up to the challenges ahead, not running away; there are no hiding places from cancer. When you face up to it head on, with a positive mind;

you respond to the situation rather than just reacting to it. Responding means you are in control and thinking about what is happening; reacting is not a controlled behaviour, reactions only giving you a short term fix and long term headaches.

Now I am in control of the things I can control, I can now fully concentrate on my trusted medical team and my outcome. I cannot control my cancer, therefore I am not going to worry; my body needs all of its strength to take on the chemotherapy treatment and any further surgery after that. I am not going to worry, and give respect to the cancer that has taken up residency in my body, that it is demanding from me. Not a chance; it's like a school bully who needs the attention to thrive; school bullies do not deserve respect, and neither does cancer. It may try to break me physically; mentally it does not have a chance.

I can handle the pain and discomfort I am facing, that is a small price to pay to spend many more years with my family and friends, pain will only be temporary, my family is for life.

Each day through treatment may be painful and hurt; however it is one day closer to the end of the cancer inside of me; closer to my finishing line, I just hope it is hurting it more than it is hurting me.

There are enough pressures placed on us for having cancer in today's modern society, we have all these confusing and conflicting messages constantly bombarding us from various media, we are left feeling guilty, confused, frustrated, and angry, emotionally drained and not in touch with ourselves, having no control over our responses to a very stressful time in our lives.

One step behind the heels of feeling powerless for having cancer; guilt strides proudly along, an evil, disguised as a kindly friend. Guilt can be described as a sense of regret or lack of responsibility. Feeling guilty over things we actually did wrong, things we believe were our fault, or things we had no responsibility for. Guilt encourages you from the side lines of cancer, giving you a false sense of security, once you accept feeling guilty and start blaming yourself for having cancer, you will find that it will drag your mind and body down even lower than before.

Accept you have cancer and make peace with yourself; don't waste energy beating yourself up and keep it in reserve for the journey ahead. No one has said to me it is going to be easy, and I am not expecting to be, I can though try making the best out of a bad situation.

Look after your mind, take control of what you can control and focus on the outcome you want; don't ever feel guilty for having cancer. Taking control is great; however, know your limitations and ask for help when needed. Courage is not just about standing up and speaking out, it is also about being able to sit down and listen.

I have set myself firm dates as land marks in my recovery.

- End of my chemotherapy treatment
- The PET Scan to see how well its worked
- The operation to remove the cancer
- The completion of my recovery programme; the finish line

August 20ᵗʰ CT Scan at Harrogate Hospital

A CT scan is special X-ray tests that produce cross-sectional images of the body using X-rays and a computer. The CT scan can help my medical team to see small nodules or tumours, which they cannot see with a plain film X-ray. CT Scans make use of computer-processed combinations of many X-ray measurements taken from different angles to produce cross-sectional images of specific areas of a scanned object, allowing the medical team to see inside my body without opening me up to have a nose around to see what is going on, on the inside.

The CT scan took about 15 minutes; nothing intrusive and just a routine procedure. When I arrived at the Hospital, I had to change my clothing into hospital gowns and was given a jug of special liquid to drink, about 5 glasses full, 30 minutes before the actual scan itself; the liquid was to highlight the my gut area and to make it easier to show up on the X ray. I also was given an x ray dye (contrast) into the vein in my right arm. This dye highlights the blood vessels and organs more clearly on the X-rays; this was administered through a cannula.

To be fair, the CT scan was very uneventful; I just lay there whilst the CT Scanning machine moved up and down my body, whirling away taking lots of images of my body.

It would be two weeks before the results would be ready; so I got dressed and went home, easy and as simple as that.

September 4th Diagnosis Results

I received a letter asking to go to Harrogate Hospital as they now have all my results from the Endoscopy, Biopsies and the CT scan. Was I feeling nervous or apprehensive was I expecting a different outcome to the one I had resigned myself to; No, I was not? This would only confirm what I already knew and in my mind, to what extent the cancer had spread and what the medical team were proposing. Dr L and a Macmillan Nurse specialist where there and went through the results; yes it was cancer and they were happy it had not spread to any other organs or lymph nodes, it was localised in my lower oesophagus, just above the stomach. So that was at least some good news that came out of the bad.

Any day to receive news that you have cancer is not good; when I was flying out to Italy the very next day for my daughter's wedding, it really sucked, timing could not have been worse. Was the cancer bothered by the timing? No, that is what it does, hits you when you least expect it and tries to bring you down, ruining any happiness that you have. Okay, it is what it is, I will deal with it; I am not going to have this spoil my daughter's wedding. Since the endoscopy, I had accepted the fact I had cancer, so maybe that's why it didn't come as a shock or too much of a surprise; I had already conditioned myself to the news.

We ran through a lot of the medical information of the results; and the Macmillan Nurse P, made notes from what the Doctor had said.

Once the Doctor had left; Nurse P gave me a whole host of information about cancer, support groups and help available to me if I needed support. The information was very good and that is why I mentioned earlier, there is no need to trawl the internet and become a keyboard Doctor. The medical team ensure you are fully up to speed on everything, keeping you well informed and constantly handing information to you.

When I left the Hospital, I did feel a little bit empty inside; my thoughts turned to my wife and children; how do I tell them this news, how would they take it, do I water it down or do I give it the worst case scenario. I had time to reflect on my way home; if I am not positive about this, how on earth can I expect them to be positive, they will respond to how I present it. The major issue for me was, I had a wedding to attend, I was going to give my daughter away, as father of the bride I had to make a speech; this was the most important thing at this moment in time for me.

I made the decision, not until after the wedding, will it become common knowledge between families and very close friends. Yes it will be hard to keep it quiet, hiding a secret that in some way would affect each and every one of them at the wedding. My cancer would have to be put on a backburner for now; even though it would be kicking and screaming in the back of my mind to get out and announce itself to all present.

It was tough to keep it hidden during the wedding weekend, especially during my wedding speech. At the part where I mentioned, "it is an honour for a father to walk their daughter down the aisle and I am very privileged to be able to fulfil that role today" BANG, wow, I had uncontrolled images and thoughts that I may not be around to walk my youngest daughter down the aisle. This really hit me out of nowhere; again, like I felt on the recovery ward, all these eyes were staring at me. Regaining composure, I got through the speech; slightly more emotional than I wanted, at least the guests thought it was just the occasion and a fathers love and happiness for their daughter on her special day.

Inside I felt drained and empty, this news of cancer was still very raw and not processed in my mind, so much so, I mentioned to my great friend Steve as the wedding photographer snapped away on her cameras. "If I am not around to walk Claire down the Aisle, I want you to do that for me; I will write the speech, I want you to do me the honour" I think this got the better of him too.

The next day after the wedding; I decided that my mind has to be stronger than my emotions; it is the only way I am going to get through this. I am not going to be viewed as a survivor of cancer or have a victim mentality, another number on the statistics chart; I am going to recover from my illness and be a normal human being without being labelled; I will walk my youngest daughter down the aisle, fit and well. "Sorry Steve, you've been stood down from your stand in father duties"

Now the excitement of the wedding day was over; we were, as a group to spend the next couple of days in each other's company. Sitting by the infinity pool contemplating in silence high up in the Italian interior mountainside, looking out across the beautiful country side, with unobstructed views, my mind wandered freely to find the best way forward from here.

As a young 16 year old, I joined Her Majesty's Royal Marine Commandos, an elite fighting force, highly regarded and respected across the world. One of their mantras which were ringing loud for me was; "Taking the impossible and making it possible- It is a State of Mind" this could not be truer at this moment in time. This cancer I have is just as much about my mental strength as it is physical; the emotions have to go, my mind has to be stronger than my emotions, otherwise my daily journey would be like my wedding speech, an emotional wreck. The four elements of a Royal Marines Commando Spirit; courage, determination, unselfishness, and cheerfulness in the face of adversity; this is even etched on the back of my wrist watch.

It was this moment I knew, I had to control this situation and not the other way around; I will control how my mind will deal with this and what information, advice I will take on board. A difficult situation does not mean it is impossible; I promised myself, I will not be afraid of what could go wrong, and remain focused about what is going to go right. I will walk my daughter down the aisle and I will spend many more years with my wife and family.

At lesson learned in life from my time in the Royal Marines; when you join the Royal Marines, they deconstruct you and rebuild you into a mentally strong individual that can cope with the hard knocks in life, the setbacks, they call it dislocated expectations; when things don't go to plan, you are well prepared mentally, physically to adapt to any situation facing you and conquer it.

The Royal Marines push you both physically and mentally beyond the limits you could ever imagine on a daily basis; even when your body is screaming to give up, your mind is disciplined and conditioned to overcome the physical pain you are enduring to get you through whatever it is you are doing. Every run, endurance course or exercise you do, you finish on a country lane that arrives to the entrance of Lympstone Barracks in Exeter, the home of training for the Marines. 500 metres from the finish, there is a tree with a large cartoon of Royal Marine character, running and giving everything he has got left in his tank to get to the end; the painted caption states on it "it is only pain". That is how I am taking my treatment; it is only pain and it will soon pass, it is not forever; it really is mind over matter.

I needed to rely on my past experiences and training; this is what is going to help me get through this. Cancer has a sole purpose to exist; to silently destroy my body and mind. If I give in to cancer and could see the impact of negative thoughts beforehand, I guarantee, I would never have them.

Cancer is a hidden disease; just because you cannot see it, it does not mean a person is not suffering inside. Please do not judge or assume anything about a person who has cancer; we have no idea what they are going through and some of that well intended advice can cause more harm than good. When talking to a person who is going through cancer, do so with the intention of leaving them in a better place mentally than when you first met them.

Listen to understand and not just to reply; tales of woe and victory are not always what people want to hear; it is their journey walk in step with them, and to their tune. Cancer sufferers are going through far more than you can imagine; please allow them the space and time to process what is happening to them; this is very important as changes to their body is constantly happening; sometimes it can be quite scary for them.

Like in the Royal Marines, do not deconstruct another person unless you are prepared to help rebuild them to something better.

"It is a state of Mind"

It is essential I have control of my emotions; otherwise the cancer will control them and use them against me. If I avoid facing up to cancer to keep the peace in my mind, Cancer will start a war inside me.

September 9th Phone call from Dr B

We arrived back in Manchester airport from Italy, and found our car in the car park, said our good byes to some of our family and friends who had caught the same return flight as us.

We were making good journey time along the M62 and the conversation was all about the wedding and the fantastic weekend we had all shared. In the car was myself driving, Fatima in the front passenger seat and Claire and Sam (Claire's long-time boyfriend) in the back. My phone rang into life, which was connected to the car Bluetooth, so whatever the conversation, it came through the car speakers for all to hear. It was Dr B; now I could have muted the call or said I would call back later, this in itself would have raised suspicions. I let the call continue; one eye on the road and one on my rear view mirror, watching Claire and Sam in the back. Dr B obviously revealed most of my situation; silenced filled the car, the shock to them both must had stunned them into complete silence. When the brief call had finished, which felt like an eternity, I said, "Yes I have cancer". There were a few tears, how quickly people can get knocked off a high moment and come crashing back down to earth.

This was not the way I wanted to break the news; I guess it was as good a time as any. The most important thing for me was how I responded to this breaking news; if I had broken down, then they would have copied, if I was positive and focused on a great outcome, then they would to; they would follow my example.

I had at this time removed the emotion out of the situation and explained it in a more logical, calculated and rational way.

The rest of the journey was very muted as one would expect; my thoughts though were focused on Simone and Wesley; news always has a way of filtering out and this is not the way I want them both to find out.

When we arrived home, I phoned Wesley and explained it to him; he responded with surprise and taken aback; at least he had heard from me. Simone was driving back from Italy through Europe with James her new husband. I messaged Simone when they had reached France and waiting to catch the ferry back across to England. She was shocked, however she told me off for not saying anything to her beforehand at the wedding.

This is now when I really accepted I have cancer; I felt at peace with myself, not harbouring a secret anymore. This was the best I felt mentally, more in control and free to get on with life as normal as possible.

Speaking to right people and not broadcasting the news, helped me maintain my thoughts and remain in a positive mental frame of mind

September 10th Appointment with the Dietician

The following day after arriving back home, I had a hospital appointment with the dietician.

A number of changes physically were happening to me and now having cancer, they made sense as to why.

- Loss of weighted, I had shed close to a stone in weight; I put it down to a very healthy diet when travelling with work. No snacking, no bread, eating mainly healthy grains, pulses, and beans. I have to admit, I feel really good with the weight off; there could have been a better reason for losing it though.
- Fatigue, this was a big one for me, I could fall asleep at any time, with a complete feeling of exhaustion that would come on at any time without warning. This I found a constant daily battle; the tiredness did affect my concentration as well.

The dietician explained that they need to stabilise my weight and not to lose anymore; I needed to calorie load so my body would be strong enough to withstand chemotherapy and surgery. I was advised to eat smaller portions more often rather than large meals; to chew my food more to help with digestion. I normally eat quickly, this comes from my days in the military; to help slow this down and eat smaller amounts, I used a cake fork; this really did the trick for me.

I needed to keep the calories in me whilst I still had an appetite and able to swallow; when I was given some examples of what to add on a daily basis to my diet, I had a smile on my face. I liked this; Mini pork pie/pasty/ packet of crisp/slice of pizza/ chocolate bar/ slice of sponge cake; all the naughty foods we are told to get rid of. There are a lot more of these tasty treats recommended, too many to list. Joking aside; they are recommended for a purpose and essential for maintaining a healthy enough body weight so my body can take the effects of what I was about to face shortly.

My weight has stabilised now which is good news; every visit to the hospital you get weighed, bloods taken, pulse and temperature all recorded; this is how serious they take your diet when having cancer. Please use and follow the dietician's advice, it is an essential part of my treatment; and as I mentioned in the beginning; my side of the deal is to follow the instructions given by the medical team; and that is what I am doing.

The dietician and all the medical teams know when you are in the hospital; even if you do not have an appointment with a specific person; they track you like air traffic control track aircraft; they know exactly where you are in the system. The reason for this is, everyone is kept up to date with your progress and if they need to see you quickly, they will come and find you whilst you are there rather than making appointment after appointment and trying to simplify life for me.

September 11th PET scan at St. James Hospital Leeds

Today was the day I had a PET scan; the reason behind this, was to give the specialists a greater and more detailed view of the inside of my organs; this was to double check that the cancer had not spread.

A PET scan (positron emission tomography) is an imaging test that allows my medical team to check for diseases in your body. They use a special dye containing radioactive tracers. These tracers were injected into a vein in arm; I believe depending on what part of the body is being examined there are different methods. Cancer cells pick up a lot of the tracers; they tend to use more energy than healthy cells. The PET scan show where the radioactive substance is in your body, slightly different to a CT scan takes pictures of the inside of the body using x-rays taken from different angles.

I was injected with the tracer and left for about an hour for it to work its way through the body; I could picture myself like a glow worm inside, toxic and radioactive, shining brightly.

The PET scan lasted about another 40 minutes, a full body scan. The machine whirled away and did its thing as I was passed through the machine, taking imagines of my entire body; it felt as if I was continually sliding through a giant Hi Tech polo mint.

When the scan had finished, I was advised to get dressed, and to use a specific bathroom away from the general public.

My results from the scan would be discussed by the multi-disciplinary medical team who were looking after me; these experts meet once a week when they have all the information available to them, then carefully plan the treatment best suited for your situation.

I have mentioned before, treatment is very specific to you and not a one size fits all; hence the reason for limiting the amount of information you take in from outside. The multi-disciplinary teams are highly trained, exceptionally talented and only work in your best interests.

September 17th Diagnosis Results

I was driving along the A1 to Newcastle for work when my phone rang. It was Nurse M, a MacMillan nurse from Harrogate Hospital.

Nurse M discussed the results with me and confirmed that the cancer was localised to the oesophagus just above the stomach. This came as good news for me; this meant it would hopefully be easier to treat and better odds stacked in my favour.

Nurse M explained the next steps for me and appointments had already been made for them and mentioned that the Multi-disciplinary team were happy with the results as well.

The next steps would be as follows:

- September 19th CPEX at LGI (heart and lung fitness Assessment)

- September 24th first meeting with the surgeon Mr s and Oncologist Consultant Dr U St James Hospital Leeds

The conversation ended on a high from the news just given and received, I continued my day as normal; it was a relief to have some concrete answers and being able to concentrate on other important things in my life.

September 19th CPEX at LGI (heart and lung fitness Assessment)

A Cardiopulmonary Exercise Testing is a non-invasive method used to assess the performance of the heart and lungs at rest and during exercise.

During the test I will be required to perform a mild exercise on an upright bicycle whilst breathing through a mouthpiece and being wired up to a monitor. Every breath of mine will be measured to assess how my body is performing. The capacity and strength of my lungs is measured before and during exercise. The heart tracing (ECG) will also be recorded prior to, during and post exercise. This builds up a picture of my body's fitness and strength to understand if it is healthy enough to withstand the treatment of chemotherapy and surgery; it will also help the medical team, decided on which chemotherapy and surgery is best in relation to my results

The test will lasted for about total of 30 minutes; some people may require less; it is not about who is fitter than who, a competition to get on to the UK cycling team; although there are people warming up in the waiting area before they go in. The test requires my maximum effort to ensure the most reliable diagnostic information is obtained, so the best treatment for me can be given. My legs gave out before my lungs as the resistance was increased on the bicycle; I was fairly pleased with my efforts although I was not exactly sure what was required; I guess those long daily dog walks helped me along the way. Wiping the perspiration off my brow and a quick glass of water; I went on my way, It still felt that I was using muscles I didn't know I had, legs feeling tight, trying hard to walk normal; probably making it look worse. Vanity

September 24ᵗʰ first meeting with the surgeon Mr S and Oncologist Consultant Dr U St James Hospital Leeds

All of my medical notes had now been transferred over to St James Hospital in Leeds; a huge specialist teaching Hospital; these now would take responsibility for my care. I would agree that it make perfect sense to have everything under one roof so to speak.

I met Mr S, the surgeon; he examined my stomach to make sure he could perform the operation when the time came for him to practice his knife wielding skills. Mr S explained thoroughly how the procedure was going to work and what his initial plans were; obviously this would be discussed in greater detail once the chemotherapy had finished and its effect on my cancer known; a further PET scan would be required after the last chemotherapy to discover this. Basically they would cut out part of the oesophagus where the tumour was and stretch the stomach up to reattach it to the remaining part of the oesophagus; this could only happen if the tumour had stopped growing or shrunk. Mr S ran through some of the changes after surgery, relearning how to eat, being fed through a tube for a short while; if I was getting fed through a tube whilst my oesophagus healed. I could try and use that as an excuse for getting out of doing the dishes at home; I wouldn't be using plates; I wonder if my wife would fall for it. Mr S arrange for me to see the dietician straight after him, who had now taken over my care in St James. At his point in time, he wanted to know if I was happy to proceed with surgery when the time came; "definitely" was my answer which pleased him as it was sensible and the answer he wanted to hear.

I approached these two meeting as the business end of it; it starts for serious now, I have the two specialists, who ultimately were responsible for my care; I was now under their expert knowledge, skills and experience. They basically had my life in their hands. "No Pressure Gentlemen; I am now putting all my faith in you both as you have the means to get rid of this cancer inside me" was the polite message I gave them. I have to be honest, both Mr S and Dr U filled me with confidence, as Mr S mentioned, "We can cure this and cut it out" music to my ears

Next I met Dr T who was Dr U (Registrar) who ran through the finer details of my treatment with chemotherapy. What the treatment they had decided on and why this particular one; what to expect from the treatment and possible side effects I was likely to incur along the way. Loss of hair; Dr T did mention, if I wanted to dye it purple, now is the opportunity before it all falls out. There were a number of very serious issues discussed about the chemotherapy and immediate action that needs to be taken if any of them happen. As mentioned earlier; it is serious from now on in; I do not underestimate cancer; I also do not underestimate the inner strength I have to not be afraid of it either. Before leaving with information sheets, Dr U popped in and introduced himself; quietly spoken man, and held in very high regard within the medical teams he works.

October 1st Sign Consent forms and decontamination wash

Although I had agreed to go ahead with treatment; chemotherapy and surgery; the hospital gave me some breathing time to go away and think about it. There is so much information to take in and absorb, to understand how this all works and the journey I am about to embark on. Obviously I discussed it with my wife and family, as they needed to have a complete grasp of the situation; they are part of this whole journey from start to finish. Involving them completely, for me, was the best thing I could do; there are no awkward moments or questions; the main thing is, we are moving forward together. It does not matter if they are small steps, as long as they are forward; progress is then being made.

I met Dr U who covered in detail the treatment plan for me, why it was this plan that was deemed the most appropriate and the results he was looking for at the end of chemotherapy. Dr U carefully explained what to expect, the highs and lows, so I was fully aware of what would be happening in a couple of weeks. He also explained that they can adjust the doses of chemotherapy and that I must not suffer in silence if it becomes too much. As with all of these things, the treatment being very personal to me; we don't know until we start how my body is going to react. From my point, there was not a great deal I could ask at this stage; the written and verbal information I had received from the start was excellent, this kept me well informed, without becoming overwhelming for me. All of the information is explained in layman terms and no question is a silly question for them.

I mentioned to Dr U, that I was quite happy and I am sure as the treatment progresses, more questions would arise which will be appropriate at the time. To that, I signed the consent form to proceed; would it be wrong to say I felt a little excited; I just want to get rid of this cancerous tumour which had taken up residency in my oesophagus, without permission and feeding off my healthy cells for free. Yes I was excited and no it isn't wrong; I don't want to wait too long to have the best for myself and I believe with Mr S and Dr U, along with their teams, I have the best

After leaving Dr U, I was then handed to a Macmillan nurse; who took a number of swabs from various parts of my body where infections can hide and grow; like MRSA. From here I was given a bottle of pink decontamination shower wash and a tube of ointment which was to be applied to the inside of my nose. I was to shower using the decontamination wash for five days before the insertion of my PICC Lines; its purpose is to do what the name describes, to decontaminate the body. The ointment was to be rubbed inside my nose, three times per day, for five days; again, this is to kill any bacteria entering through my nostrils.

It was now time to wait for my next three appointments; these will be confirmed very soon by post and will include; a pre op assessment and visit to the oncology ward on the first appointment.

For my second appointment I will have the insertion of the PICC Lines, these will remain in my arm for the duration of the entire chemotherapy treatment.

My third appointment will be the start of the chemotherapy itself.

I have had numerous visits to St James Hospital in the large modern cancer wing. Is it a depressing place? No it isn't; it is very relaxed, caring and efficient place to be, with outstanding staff and people who care as much about you as you do about you.

You guys do an amazing job and are often underappreciated; certainly not from me, my family, my friends and the many other people I have met during my time with you, in your care.

October 7th Pre Assessment for Chemotherapy

I arrived at the hospital for my pre-arranged appointment; my height, weight, bloods and pulse were taken again as they want to monitor any changes in my circumstances.

From here I went through to see Senior Nurse J; at this point he went through what the process of treatment that had been specifically tailored for my condition and needs. I was after each chemotherapy session at the Hospital to have chemotherapy pump attached to my PICC Lines; this was to give me another 24 hours of chemotherapy at home. I was shown how it would be attached and how the pump worked, what to look out for, what to do and not to do; After the 24 hours the pump had been running, a district nurse would come to my home address and disconnect the pump, clean the area and put a clean dressing on. I would be in regular contact to see the nurse, generally every

Friday. Whilst Nurse J was going through the information; he asked if I was on any supplements, vitamin tablets, drinks etc. I had not even thought about this; apparently certain vitamin tablets react badly to chemotherapy and should not be taken at all whilst on treatment. Nurse J listed the supplements I was taken and sent them to the hospital pharmacists for analysis; these I decided to stop taking there and then. The time of year it is now, it is time for flu jabs; again there are certain times when I can take flu jab during chemotherapy treatment; I was advised to have it about two days before my next treatment as this is when my immune system would have recovered to its strongest and be able to tolerate it.

There is so much information that needs to be taken in from the cancer specialists; again I cannot reiterate how much I really needed to listen and fully understand what they are telling me; it is not generic information; it is information specific to me. I know I am beating the drum about listening to everyone on the outside telling me what I can and can't do, what I should and shouldn't do; with all the good intentions meant; it is muddying the waters and having a reverse affect to what you are trying to achieve. Cancer is a very personal journey; and it is a journey that needs a clear outcome and process to reach that outcome

From here, Nurse J showed me around the oncology ward, where the reception was, where the treatment was going to take place and an over view of the day that was planned for me. This short tour but, a very vital tour that was enough to get my head around the treatment that I was going to have administered on this ward in a few days' time. As part of the tour, we also looked at where the PICC Lines will be inserted; all this is done to put my mind at ease and to reduce any unnecessary stress and anxiety that I may have.

From here I was given some steroid tablets to take home, I was to have 4 the morning prior to my treatment and 4 on the morning of my treatment.

October 9th PICC Lines get inserted

I was called through to a mini theatre to have the PICC lines inserted; as normal all my details are checked and cross checked. I was introduced to the medical staffs that were going to insert the lines and how it was going to be done.

A PICC line is most often used to deliver medication over a long period. The nurse will insert the PICC line, which is a thin tube, into a vein in the arm. The tube is advanced until it reaches the superior vena cava, a vein that carries blood to the heart, in my case this was 48 cm in length.

When they insert it, they have a little monitor to track the line; if they are happy with the positioning of the line they fix it in place and that then remains there for the entire time of my treatment. If they cannot track the line, then I would need an x ray to check that is positioned correctly.

I lay on the bed so they could prepare me for the line insertion; I had my right arm stretch out to the side as they prepared it, whilst another nurse began to attach the probe pads to my shoulders; two were put on my shoulders and two on my hips. My arm was being cleaned and although I could not see properly, there where large amounts of plastic sheets being placed across my arm; part of the sheeting was lying across my chest and side of my face. The nurse said she would move it just now; they need the sheets to prevent cross contamination; I replied "phew, I thought you were getting my body bag ready" this brought a chuckle to proceeding. Laughter is a great medicine; if you are laughing and it's not working, then laugh some more.

The procedure began; the most painful bit for me was probably the anaesthetic needle, which is not painful at all, just like any other injection. The procedure itself did not take too long, about 10/15 minutes and fortunately for me, the line could be traced and an x ray was not needed.

Once cleaned up, I was given information on how to look after the lines to prevent damage to them and advice if I need any help or have any concerns. I was given a card to carry at all times in case of emergencies to warn any medical staff who assisted me, that I am on chemotherapy and the need for them to take the correct safety precautions and what to administer and what not to. This card also contains emergency numbers which are manned 24 hours per day; they cannot overstate that I must call it any time of the day or night, with any concerns, especially, bleeding, high temperature and feeling unwell.

Before leaving the Nurse gave me a shopping bag of medical equipment and dressing for the district nurse to use and safely dispose of the pump and dressings; these are very toxic from the chemotherapy and needed handling with care.

October 10th, Chemotherapy Cycle One, and following days.

My first cycle started today, I felt a little apprehensive. The information I had been given thus far was fantastic; still there is always the unknown.

The schedule of treatment for me contains four drugs: three are chemotherapy-Docetaxel, Oxaliplatin and Fluorourcil. The fourth is Calcium Folinate. The regime I will be given; a drip of Docetaxel followed by a drip of Oxaliplatin at the same time as a drip of Calcium Folinate. I would then receive Fluorourcil for 24 hours by a pump at home. This treatment is known as FLOT for short.

I sat on a chair and my PICC Line was flushed to remove any debris and dried blood; the insertion wound was also cleaned before we could begin. I was asked if I had taken any supplements as these can interfere with the chemotherapy and if I had taken my steroid tablets yesterday and today. At every stage, my details are checked, crossed checked and before any drug is administered, checked by two nurses who check the product, the product code and date, the amount of the product and the speed it has to be administered; their attention to detail is second to none. Before starting the chemotherapy I had a drip which had anti -histamine and anti-sickness medication to help me tolerate the treatment better and was told it really works to reduce nausea; all of these are fed through the PICC Lines. These took about 3 hours to complete and then I was ready for the chemotherapy itself; these come up in thick black plastic bags to avoid any contact with light sources; even when on the drip stand it is covered with the black bag; apparently the light can reduce the chemotherapy effectiveness if exposed for long periods of time during an infusion. In total my day on the ward lasted just over six hours; a very long day, but essential. Six hours is a long time to be sitting in a chair gazing into space. In one of the information leaflets I remember reading that hypnotherapy or meditation is good for you; fortunately I am trained in these two disciplines so set about it; the peacefulness and living in the moment whilst nurses busied themselves attending to everyone, blocking out the noise was blissful; I knew those skills would come in handy sometime to use on me. Hearing other patients around me, i found it fascinating, their stories and listening to the nurses, I learned so much from quietly sitting there and listening. I keep going back to it, it is a personal journey and one size does not fit all; your treatment is for specifically for you and nobody else except the experts who are delivering it on the ward. Cancer is a very complicated and complex disease that affects each individual differently, and there are so, so many different forms of cancer out there. We have one thing in common though, to rid ourselves of this disease through a cocktail of toxic chemotherapy infusion.

There are people at a different stage in their treatment; it was my first session, so did not what to bring or what not to; to keep myself amused during this period. The people who have been through this before and are further down the road to recovery, they know where everything is and have come armed and prepared with electronic devices to do work or entertain themselves. I will know better next time, however, I have to admit, the relaxation and quietness was lovely.

Once the chemotherapy drip was finished, I was given a various medicines to take home, anti-sickness tablets, diarrhoea sachets to bung you up and medication to take before the next round of chemotherapy; steroids and more anti-sickness tablets.

I had the chemotherapy pump attached to the PICC Lines which was to use to administer another 24 hours of chemotherapy at home; This chemotherapy was the Fluorouracil; this will be disconnected by the district nurse after that 24 hour period. All this is pre-arranged for you, so there is no need to worry about the admin side of things, that is all taken care of for me, my focus is on recovery

Today I have woken up and feel ok, nauseous; the anti-sickness drug appears to be keeping everything in; I took one last night before bed and one this morning as advised to do, not just by the medical teams, but by other patients who had regretted not doing it, and learned a very hard lesson.

To be fair, the treatment has been manageable, maybe the side effects get worse as I proceed through the treatment and my immune system runs down and the body weakens through the chemotherapy; my mind won't weaken, it is only pain and won't last.

I have just noticed as I am sitting here, that I am getting pins and needles in the tips of my fingers, I was told this would happen and it would be become awkward to do up buttons;

tie shoe laces; it will soon pass, at least I know the chemotherapy is doing the rounds of my body, patrolling it to destroy the tumour hiding inside of me.

The chemotherapy pump was removed late yesterday afternoon by the district nurse, Nurse L, a very calm, reassuring, modern day Florence Nightingale; Nurse L just oozed kindness and care. The entire contents of the pump have to be empty, to ensure the maximum dosage that has been prescribed has entered my system. The procedure was straight forward enough; lots of sterilisation and flushes being pushed through the tube where the chemotherapy is fed; the whole thing took about half an hour and painless.

I woke up this morning, day 2; no change for the better or worse. The feeling of tiredness and being nauseous has remained the same; feeling really tired though as I was up to the loo during the night about 5 times. I have to say, I am not too bad and feel better moving around rather than just sitting still. I am not too sure how I should be feeling, should I be reeling in pain, bed ridden, projectile vomiting, I honestly don't know. Side effects of chemotherapy affect each individual differently; everyone reacts in a different way to treatment, so it's hard to say how I might feel. Some people might struggle with side effects, while others sail through. I try to remember that, although the side effects of cancer treatment can be tough, most of them are only short-term and will gradually disappear once my cycle of chemotherapy treatment is completed. The one thing I have noticed is being constipated; this is quite uncomfortable. Hopefully after a few large glasses of prune juice I have just drank, that should get the insides moving and back in working order.

The prune juice has done it thing, the bloating of my stomach has appeared to ease somewhat; it feels so much better today, not perfect, but that pain and discomfort is more manageable. I have decided that just before my next chemotherapy session and for the couple of days after it, I will eat softer foods like soups which are far easier to digest and less likely to bung me up. I guess it's a bit of trial and error on what to eat and what not to, to help prevent constipation; and disgusting as it is, a glass of prune juice daily will help keep me regular.

Today (3) is it the last day for taking my anti sickness tablets; I have to take 2 tablets, twice a day for three days. I can take them now as and when required; I am interested to see how I get on without them. I have noticed that my jaw has become painful when starting to eat; it wears off very quickly; after 30 seconds or so and then it's back to normal again. There is a whole list of side effects that could potentially come my way;

- Bruising and Bleeding from the gums
- Anaemia
- Sickness
- Diarrhoea
- Hair Loss

- Sore mouth
- Tiredness and Fatigue
- Joint Pain

There are more listed for you and you are expected to get some if not all of them. There are some that need immediate medical attention like heart and breathing problems; sometimes the treatment can affect your breathing, heart and lungs which can potentially be life threatening. These are signs that I need to be aware off so appropriate action can be swift.

Having a healthy positive mind will help you through these; try not to over think every little discomfort and make it an all or nothing scenario. Yes the side effects need to be monitored, but in a controlled manner; try not to let your imagination run wild; especially in the dark of the night when nobody is around to talk to.

Day (4); it has been 24 hours since taking my last anti sickness tablet, at this particular moment in time; I do not feel a need to have any. The bloating and constipation has eased to a more comfortable and manageable level.

The one curious thing I have noticed; where I have had previous operations like a broken leg, hernias and old injuries, there appears to be a dull ache around those trauma areas. This is not painful, just more of an observation than anything. Other than this, I am feeling reasonably okay and happy to try and go back to work; albeit on lighter duties, even part time. This I will have to monitor and keep everything in balance.

One of the side effects from most cancer treatments results in hair loss; this can whole body, including eyelashes, eye brows and total body hair. Sometimes it may just be confined to loss of hair from one's head; the hair loss tends to start after week three of treatment.

A little victory for me today; I cut my hair extremely short, in barber speak, a grade one. I am not going to allow cancer the pleasure to have my hair fall out when it wants; I cut it on my terms and how I wanted; any hair loss after this would be minimal and people would probably not notice. This may sound petty or silly; however, it put a small smile on my face as I could deny cancer all the fun it wanted at my expense.

Having a positive mind and being around positive people is very good for your health; I honestly love it. I will not end up as another one of life's tragedies. Being in the company of positive people, you are not judged, there is no drama and everyone just wants to be happy, relaxed, and focused to deal with the situation they face. I hope that by reading this book, you will take the same path; believe in yourself, surround yourself with positive people and know you can achieve anything.

I have made a few changes to diet and daily routine; these have had a positive impact on me, and even though they may be small impacts, the cumulative effect will be greater:

- I have stopped drinking tea and coffee; for me I found that it made me feel nauseous about 30 minutes after drinking
- I have stopped drinking any fizzy drink; I don't drink much of this stuff anyway, but thought an energy drink would help. Like the tea and coffee, it again made me feel nauseous and quite painful as it moved down my oesophagus.
- I make sure any food I am eating is not too hot and has had time to cool sufficiently; again like the fizzy drink, it made me feel nauseous and quite painful as it moved down my oesophagus.
- If I feel tired, unwell or need some peace and quiet, I find it more beneficial to lie down rather than just sit in an arm chair. It appears to take any pressure off my oesophagus and relieve any discomfort.
- I have started to walk a bit more now as well to remain active; not too far but enough to get the heart rate going; it is also more mentally stimulating than

watching day time TV. It is important that I have wrapped up well with scarf and hat, now is not the time to get an infection or an illness that could set me back any further.

As with all of these things, I am learning as I go along; trial and error; anything that helps me from talking to god on the big white telephone, must be helping. I will try and prepare myself better for the next session of chemotherapy; to help stave off constipation and pass the time at the hospital

I always keep in mind when I do feel rough and having a bad day; that there are many other people out there who are suffering or worse off than me; many of those are suffering in silence. My pain and discomfort is insignificant compared to their plights; and in many circumstances, they do not have the professional help like the NHS to get them through it.

Cancer wants me to complain about my pain and discomfort, to feel sorry for myself; that is what it does; it feeds off my suffering and distress, running my health into the ground even further.

I have made a promised to myself that I will never complain and let cancer get the better of me; it is not getting any recognition from me that will help it grow and become stronger. This is what it craves, it wants to boost its own ego and force me into submission; the one thing it hasn't taken into consideration is my stubbornness and will to survive.

Life will not always deal me a great hand; that is just the way it goes. The most important thing is how I respond to the situation; that response will go a long way to determining the outcome. Understanding my body and mind at each stage of the treatment, will give me the response I need and not to just to go with the flow and have the cancer control me.

Today is one week after receiving my first chemotherapy session; I feel good today. This is the best I have felt for a long time, even before chemotherapy started; I feel healthy, with no discomfort at all; it is a great day and I am going to make the most of it. Walking the dogs through the beautiful Yorkshire countryside, fresh air and enjoying the simple pleasures that life has to offer. This is a natural medicine and stimulates the senses to give me that feel good factor, my own bodies natural defence mechanism; one giant stride for me, one step backwards for cancer.

One thing that I have noticed, which I believe to be a good sign is; with oesophagus cancer you can experience a very sharp, tight pain in the centre of the chest. This tightness and discomfort appears now to have disappeared; could this be the chemotherapy working already in breaking down the cancer cells? Has Dr U's, the cancer wizard's magic potion for me worked? I do not have any scientific proof or medical evidence to substantiate this at this stage; this is what my body is telling me, I trust those messages it is giving me.

Whatever the reason for the discomfort going, which has been there constantly for months now; it certainly is a very welcome boost of positivity to the mind. I am happy to take it for what it is and believe now that I am making progress on the road to recovery.

October 22nd Pre Assessment for Chemotherapy Cycle Two

I arrived at the hospital for my pre-arranged appointment; my height, weight, bloods and pulse were taken again as they want to monitor any changes in my circumstances. The easy thing about having my bloods taken was; they could draw the blood down through the PICC Line. This removed the need for more injections and another appointment with the haematologist. Before the blood was drawn, the PICC Line was cleaned and flushed to remove any debris that could have blocked the line. Once all the pre assessments had been completed, it took 10 minutes to do; I then had an appointment with the Doctor.

The Doctor ran through a number of questions to see how I coped with the chemotherapy and any side effects that I may have experienced. The main purpose was to ensure that the Chemotherapy dosage was correct for me by noting any physical changes or having a bad reaction to it. These changes could then be made before my second cycle of chemotherapy in two days' time. I did mention to the Doctor about the tightness in my chest easing to virtually nothing and removing food that had got stuck in my oesophagus was easily dislodged with a sip of water. She mentioned that it was more than likely not coincidence and that the chemotherapy was having an effect and it was a very positive and encouraging sign if it was the case. That concluded my visit for today; feeling really encouraged and Positive.

Having been able now to get my head around my cycles of chemotherapy and what to expect from them; I appreciate each cycle can have different effects on me should not be ignored; my main focus has now turned to the second half of my recovery programme in a couple of months; Surgery. In my own mind, this is going to be the toughest part of my recovery from cancer; it does not matter what type of surgery

Mr S opts for, which is determined by the outcome of the chemotherapy; it is a very invasive procedure. Even the keyhole surgery which is less invasive; it is still very invasive.

Following surgery I will more than likely have tubes sticking out of my body for various reasons; tubes through the nose and into the stomach to remove fluid from it, tube into the chest to remove fluid from it, tube into the small intestine for feeding, this is because there is nil by mouth for a minimum of a week and a catheter fitted to my bladder to drain away urine. I have this image of me looking like a colander which someone has emptied spaghetti into it and there are lots of strands poking out of it. I believe in some cases, the medical team will keep you asleep for a few days after surgery to aid recovery; it sounds to me a good idea for that to happen

After surgery the recovery of learning to eat again and leading a normal healthy life becomes the new challenge ahead of me. I have started to try and increase my fitness levels and take on more calories so my body can withstand the onslaught of what is coming its way. One thing for certain, I will be prepared both mentally and physically for it and then to cross my finish line.

My work requires me to travel a lot along the motorway networks of the UK. It was Interesting to be made aware of strict rules that the Health and Safety have around working whilst on chemotherapy. These rules will vary from job role to job role; some that apply to me are:

- I cannot work for a minimum of three days after a chemotherapy cycle
- If my travel time (driving) is over one hour, then I have to phone the office to say when I am setting off and when I arrive, same for the return journey
- If I travel by train, a three hour journey only and my place of work cannot be more than a fifteen minute walk away from the station. Again I have to phone

the office on leaving and arriving, same for the return journey
- I cannot work on site for more than five hours in one day
- If working from home completing administrative work, I cannot work for more than five hours in one day

There are more rules to it than just above; I know some cancers fall under the disabilities act and worker rights; however employers are hand tide by the Health and Safety Executives; it may be worth checking out what you can and cannot do whilst on your treatment.

I thought it would be down to me and how I felt at the time; obviously there is far more red tape to it than one can imagine.

When having chemotherapy and recovering from it; I have a lot of time on my hands. I find using this time for relaxing the mind and body either through self-hypnosis or meditation very beneficial to me. It helps me clear the mind, refresh my body and to relax quite deeply. The most powerful tool I have at my disposal to come through this is my mind; it is therefore essential it remains strong, de-cluttered and focused on my finish line. My mind needs to be focused only on what I have and what I want; not what I don't have and don't want, which is what cancer would like; it would put me in a negative mind frame, opening up the channels more easily for it to grow and spread. When relaxed I practice visualisation techniques of my body dealing with the cancer, healing itself; I also reflect on my journey so far and acknowledge what has been achieved already on my short journey. This I feel is really important for me; looking at the finish line constantly may seem a far off place and can at times make the journey there feel unending, a dream in the distance. Looking at what I've overcome so far, keeps the motivation going and my focus on the end point; it also allows me the satisfaction that progress is being made; does not matter how much, as long as it is being made.

I found that my recovery came in three stages as I went along. Having flexibility in my thinking on how I will deal with cancer will play a key role in me recovering from it.

Initial Plan stage; the motivation stage; the commitment stage.

- The initial thought and plan on how it going to play out for me. As I went through treatment this plan did fade for many reasons; the pain and discomfort, the change of routines, the change in personal circumstances. This will caused that initial plan to fade.
- Next I need the motivation to continue; this also faded if progress is slow and my body starts to wear down through the chemotherapy and just trying to get through one day at a time. The first two, the initial plan and motivation are conscious thoughts and easily distracted

and knocked off course when the going gets tough.

- The third part is commitment; this is the key to overcoming this disease. This is where the mind takes over and guides me from here; this is my get out of jail card that will keep me alive. This is a subconscious thought, this is what I am made of and calling on all the positive resources I have to commit to me getting through it. This is the only reserve I can truly rely on to see this through.

I have also found routine is good for me; getting up at the same time, going to bed at the same time, meals and so on. For me this allows by body clock to stay in a rhythm and reduces any unnecessary swings and changes that it constantly needs to adjust to; there is enough for it to do when the chemotherapy is fed into it. I am trying to work out what works best for me and what is not; if I try something and it does not work, I do not treat it as I have failed; I just look at it as I have found a way not to do something. These techniques work for me; if they don't work for you, try something else; it is all about keeping focused and not giving up at any stage on the journey. I have heard from some family and friends this week who, I know are being caring and trying to be kind; however, going back to the way comments are given, it can have the opposite effect of what is trying to be achieved by them. My Wife and Daughter mentioned that people are only being kind and helpful; they want to be there for me and not to push them away. That is the last thing I wish to happen, we all need support in our lives, especially in situations that are serious. I get that 100%, without question, I know people care deeply; I know people want to support me and I really do appreciate it. At this moment I need people to have empathy, to stand in my shoes, to walk in my shoes, to see the situation through my eyes, to fully understand my journey. This cannot happen if this understanding is not gained and built up on by all of us. I was in two minds to remove this piece, rather than sounding like a grumpy ungrateful person; after long deliberation I decided to leave it in. I find it far too important to be missed; a person who may not have a strong mind, who maybe suffering worse than I; whose minds are in a bad place already; things like this can cause them to give up as they are believe all hope as gone for them.

If you sit and actually read and think about the comments; from my perspective, it is going against all the positive focus I have built up in my mind. It is telling me that I have given up on trying to get well; if I survive cancer I may drop dead anyway; I cannot look to the future only one day at a time; No one can help me accept God or the church. If that is the case, should I stop treatment and just let fate run its course. Certainly not; the bells are not going to toll for me just yet, there is still life left in me to live.

"You are so brave, I could not do it" Really? I have a one way ticket to health and recovery; if I don't use it, I die-simple as that. Bravery does not come into it one bit; it is the will to survive, and do what has to be done.

"You are only feeling better because I have prayed for you" That's very kind, it really is and I really appreciate it. I do believe most of it is down to the skill of Dr U and his magic potions he pours into me very two weeks and my steely determination to get through this.

"I told you so and you need to do this and that, it is best for you" Really? What reason is it best for me?

"A friend of a friend had cancer and this happened to them and that happened to them. They died in the end; really? That was extremely positive and useful.

"You cannot look past one day at a time; do not focus on the operation; it is all in God's hands now"?? Do I not have a future? Am I not allowed to plan ahead? Do I and the medical teams not have a say in my outcome? Am I to be stripped of all my hopes and dreams? Am I just fooling myself?

Cancer is a silent destroyer of the body and mind; it will eat its way through me for one sole purpose, to kill me; that's it in a nutshell. It wants to kill me. I know very well it could do that; I am not ignoring this fact that it may take me physically at any time; the one thing it will not do, is take me mentally. I will not have any dark moments in my mind along this journey; and will remain committed to getting better. Once I have lost my dreams and hopes; I lose my mind and all else fails, there is nothing left to live for; I may as well give up now and hand cancer the freedom it wants to destroy me.

In general, I do not like being around negative people; they suck the life out of you and bring you down to their level with every breath they take. Listening constantly, to a person who has nothing constructive or positive to say can be soul destroying, tiresome and demotivating. Being in the position I find myself in at this moment in time; maybe I am on high alert or over sensitive to negativity and reading too much into things. I look at it this way; I find cancer is a sense of unease, a disease, where the ground is constantly shifting beneath my feet; where only my constant vigilance is the only hope of effectively protecting me.

Please, don't stop praying, lighting candles and being there for me; do though; stand in my shoes and see it from my perspective; after all that is the one that really matters. I just want you to join me on my journey and experience it how I do; I am fully focused, positive and motivated to see this through and will not be side stepped on my outcome. If I do not stand up to the cancer inside of me; the school bully;

or any other conflict I face; that situation will create a war inside of me. This will only help to weaken my resolve, my determination and dilute the positive thoughts I have about getting better. Not standing up and facing the situation head on, will only turn me against me and then cancer will happily continue on it path of destruction and have the freedom to do what it wishes; unopposed. I fully understand that when we sometimes do things that only benefit ourselves; it can upset other people. For me this treatment has to benefit me so it will allow me to spend more time with you all in the future. A mind is like water, when it is turbulent, it is difficult to see, and when it is calm, then everything becomes clear. I will stoically hold on to my thoughts of making more memories with my family and you all in the future. My mind will not become a tragedy to cancer and I will live my life in peace rather than just finding peace when I'm laid to rest.

After all said and done "I love you all as much today as I did yesterday; and thank you all from the bottom of my heart for being there for me and my family". It means everything

The power of the mind

Your beliefs become your thoughts
your thoughts become your words
your words become your actions
your actions become your habits
your habits become your values
your values become your destiny

October 24nd, Chemotherapy Cycle Two and following days.

Today is the day to have my second cycle of chemotherapy; knowing what lies ahead removes any nervousness or apprehension that I might have had otherwise. It also means that I will be half way through my planned chemotherapy treatment; now that has to be a feel good factor in itself; even though I will be having poison poured into my veins once again.

I am more prepared for the day; to pass the time I have an electronic reader, which also has Netflix loaded on to it, so fingers crossed the time will fly by. I also started eating softer foods and drinking more water yesterday in the hope of preventing the constipation I suffered after my last session. I have put a supply of my trusty prune juice in the fridge as a backup.

I did not have a great sleep last night, laying there just watching the clock slowly tick by until it is time to get up. For some unknown reason the theme song from the TV comedy show "Dads Army" from yester year came into my head; some of the lyrics had changed, certainly not by me consciously; I cannot get the tune out of my head now; still it puts a cheeky grin on my face. Now you have started singing it, I am sure it will be the same for you, playing on a constant loop in your head; maybe any of you musical geniuses out there could have a Christmas number one with it to raise money for cancer research. I do not follow dad's army and only knew the first line of the song; somewhere deep in my memory back, this catchy tune must have lodged itself for use in the future. I am sure stranger things in life have happened; maybe it's the medication, maybe it's just another positive mental attitude affirmation; whatever the reason, it makes me happy so I guess it doesn't really matter.

Here is the verse constantly being played in my head to the Dads Army Tune.

**Who do you think you are kidding Mr
Cancer?
If you think that I'm on the run?
I am the one who will stop your little
game.
I am the one who will make you think
again.
'Cause who do you think you are
kidding Mr Cancer.
If you think old David's done?**

I have taken the steroid tablets and anti-sickness tablet as advised before my treatment is to start today; and now I am setting off for the hospital. Daft as it may sound; I am looking forward to it, buoyed by the positive experienced my body appears to have had to the first cycle of chemotherapy.

Another long day at the hospital yesterday as I am hooked up to drips of varies drugs pouring into my system. The nurses as always are highly efficient and professional in their roles looking after us all. My day followed the same routine as last time, so no change in treatment of dosages, the schedule of treatment for me contains four drugs: three are chemotherapy-Docetaxel, Oxaliplatin and Fluorourcil. The fourth is Calcium Folinate. The regime I will be given; a drip of Docetaxel followed by a drip of Oxaliplatin at the same time as a drip of Calcium Folinate. I would then receive Fluorourcil for 24 hours by a pump at home. This will be a repeat cycle every two weeks; the dosage may change, all depending on how my body copes with it.

I had a bit off a sleepless night; I woke about 3 am with quite a sore chest; it felt as if the chemotherapy was specifically targeting the cancer cells in my oesophagus. This was quite sore and after about an hour, I was beginning to think that it may be time to call the emergency numbers they had given me as the pain did not ease; only intensified. On one hand I knew it was working away doing what it was supposed to be doing; on the other it can could be a serious side effect of the chemotherapy. I managed to shift by body position to lay more on my side, this helped relive the pain quite quickly and now I feel ok; maybe it was just the angle I had fallen asleep on and pressure in my oesophagus had built up.

After chemotherapy now, I have to keep taking two steroid tablets for two days after chemotherapy, and my anti-sickness tablets. The one positive thing I noticed; switching my diet to a soft diet of soup the day before chemotherapy and the day of chemotherapy has relived any constipation and bloating which I initially found quite uncomfortable. I still ensure I drink plenty of water and prune juice to keep me regular. These are little adjustments; however I find the benefits quite big for me and how I am feeling.

I took the dogs for a short walk with my wife for some fresh air; I mentioned that I felt a few spots of cold rain on my face; it was forecast rain soon that morning. It was not rain; it was the exposed skin on my face to the cold air. Pins and needles spread across my face, like tiny little hail stones where pinging off my cheeks; tiny little stabbing motions and cold sensations. This sensation spread across to my back and shoulders; it was sore, just a strange feeling of how the chemotherapy was working inside my body. I was aware that I could be more sensitive to cold as a side effect, so there was no need to panic; once home in the warmth it disappeared after 10 minutes and everything settled to normal.

I am experiencing the effects of being exposed to the cold temperature; this is through touch or by drinking a juice which is slightly chilled. The sensation I am getting is pins and needles in the back of my throat and hands, it not painful, just a weird sensation which I did not have on my first cycle of chemotherapy. I just need to take precautions to prevent this happening; add warm water to the juice, wear gloves and just to be mindful of my surroundings. This will soon pass once the chemotherapy wears off after the initial treatment has worked its way around the body.

My chemotherapy pump was to be removed 12 hours ago, 18.30 last night; unfortunately the Fluorouracil autoinfuser pump still had half of my the chemotherapy inside of it which has not entered my body. After speaking to the nurse; they mentioned that I leave it till morning, a further 12 hours to see if it has emptied. The chemotherapy has gone down by 100ml, however there is still the same amount left in the pump. Apparently the pumps don't always work to time and delays can be fairly common when using them. Having spoken to the hospital; they mentioned it can run safely for 48 hours before needing to be detached from my arm and the lines cleaned and flushed.

Finally my autoinfuser has now emptied; 45 hours it took, but I am happy that all the contents have gone into my system to set about destroying my cancer. The nurse has been, disconnected the pump, cleaned the lines and changed the dressing to ensure everything is safe and sterile. I do feel drained from and groggy from after this period of being hooked up; however as long as it is doing what it is supposed to do, that is what really counts in the grand scale of things.

I was thinking about my post-surgery and recovery whilst in hospital; I will be having tubes poking out of my body here, there and everywhere. To pass the time away with other patients, I could become a human form of the Ker-plunk game; pull a straw out and don't drop an organ. I could even attached one of those foil wine bags from the box to a feeding tube, a little tipple as we play Ker-Plunk that could be fun. I just found the thought quite amusing, it put a smile on my face and made me laugh out loud.

It is now day three after receiving my chemotherapy and the only difference to my first cycle is; I appear to be more prone to the excessive cold temperatures. I get pins and needles more readily from either being exposed to the cold or touching something cold. It is not a scary experience and soon passes once warm again. I think for me the hardest bit is the lack of constant sleep, my sleep is constantly broken through toilet visits or trying to get comfortable. I think it will probably help if I take on more regular naps throughout the day. I just want to keep my energy levels up as surgery is not too far away. My appetite is still healthy which is pleasing, again for surgery, along with my strength, not losing weight will play a vital part in my recovery.

I have noticed since receiving chemotherapy and steroids that there is a slight change in my mood; I appear to be more easily annoyed or frustrated by silly things that would not normally bother me one bit. Most of these annoyances are down to the medication, being constantly tired and a totally different routine which makes them slightly more difficult to deal with. It is dawning on me how much the medication I am on has an influence of nearly every aspect of my life from diet, digestion, eyesight, concentration, mood, my sleeping patterns, my fitness levels, and general well-being, what I am able to do and not do. It is a strange situation to be in; like a puppeteer controlling the puppet. One common factor I find we all deal with in having cancer is the unknown; is treatment working? What happens next? Do you ever really go into full remission or be cured? Or does cancer just lay there waiting to grab an opportunity to return, biding its time to strike when you least expect it? All these unanswered questions can cause stress and make you feel anxious; this is a situation I need to be careful about as it is not helpful in my recovery.

I Know I keep mentioning the importance of having a strong mind; keeping it clear and focused on my outcome. The reasons for me are; if my mind was allowed to slip or become infested with negativity; I believe two things will happen; I will become stressed and anxious. Neither of these two conditions is good for my mind and body, especially when I need all my reserves to see me through cancer. For me to avoid becoming stressed or anxious an understanding what the possible causes of these two conditions are and the affects they can have on me was helpful.

A feeling of stress comes from any situation in which we feel frustrated, angry or anxious. Stress is the way that we can feel when pressure is placed on us; it is our body's natural reaction to fear and change, or a perceived threat to us. At some time in our lives we will all suffer from stress, some people will be able to deal with it far better than others will, some will not be able to cope so well. Often too much stress can be a debilitating condition, with physical, mental and emotional problems. Once our stress response has been activated, it cannot be stopped until the response has completed its cycle, roughly about 15/20 minutes. Our health will pay the price if we experience everyday as an emergency, this will eventually cause our reaction or response to the stressor becoming more damaging than the stressor itself, which in my case is the cancer. "Sleep and stress have an uncomfortable relationship with each other: lack of sleep causes stress and stress causes lack of sleep"

Feelings of anxiety come from apprehension or fear, people all experience feelings of anxiety during their lifetime. We may feel worried and anxious about sitting an examination, taking a driving test, or a job interview. These feelings of anxiousness are perfectly normal and pose no threat to us. It becomes a serious issue when these feelings become much more constant and start to affect our day-to-day life. Anxiety can also be the main symptom for other disorders, panic disorder, phobias, PTSD. People who feel anxious most days will often struggle to remember when they last felt relaxed. This can cause both psychological and physical symptoms. Some people are more susceptible to feelings of anxiety than others and are able to deal with it in different ways. Anxiety can significantly affect our daily life, making it difficult to perform everyday tasks. The symptoms can often be slow to develop, and the severity will vary from person to person, this will cause a change in our behaviour and the way we think and feel about things. The down side of being continuously anxious is our subconscious mind will work overtime and will respond to all situations that feel remotely similar to the original feeling of anxiousness. Severe acute anxiety reactions can lead to panic attacks, which can be very debilitating.

Anxiety affects our whole being, our emotions, our behaviour and our health. It primarily creates a feeling of fear that makes us want to avoid situations that it is trying to get us to avoid for our own safety. Anxiety can be made worse by constantly having negative thoughts about a situation; these negative thoughts will compound the feelings of fear and therefore become a precursor for depression. Anxiety feeds anxiety- it continually feeds itself.

Facing up to the situation I find myself in, controlling my emotions, what I will accept and what I will not accept; will help me remove the stress and anxiety from the situation. It keeps me in control of the things I can control; I do not wish to burden myself with more unnecessary pressures than I already have; unnecessary pressures I would not have control of. Being stressed or anxious in my case would be counterproductive to my outcome and would just place more barriers in the way towards my finish line.

Having family and friends who have empathy about my situation is a huge benefit to reducing stress and anxiety; it allows for me to talk without trying to explain every detail and a feeling of not being judged. When family and friends have empathy, everyone is on the same page, all moving in the same direction with a common understanding of what the goal is. When I have felt frustrated, I have also quietly taken myself off, removed myself from the situation as not to affect anyone else and to gather my thoughts and composure. I find this quite useful and defuse any potential awkward situations that could possibly arise from my moods. The last thing I would wish is to offend anyone, turn away their kindness; once a word has been spoken in anger, it can never be undone.

Day four after my second cycle of chemotherapy and apart from feeling tired, I am not too bad. A lot of the aches and pains have subsided; nausea has reduced to a comfortable level; this in itself is a boost to my moral as a sense of normality resumes.

I have noticed today that a few hairs have starting to fall from my head; this is quite normal from the information I was given about my treatment. This is more likely to happen within the second cycle of chemotherapy as it also destroys the good cells along with the cancerous cells. Once chemotherapy has finished, my hair will grow back; like with my pain, hair loss in this case is only temporary; as it is around Christmas time now, I could find temporary work in a Christmas Grotto as a giant shiny bauble.

I am sitting looking out into the garden; it is autumn now and the bright colours of the leaves falling from the trees look spectacular, bright reds, oranges and yellows. As the leaves settle on the ground, it covers it in nature's natural golden blanket. If you are feeling low and all is lost, battling through your darkest hours, keep in mind; you will grow back just as the leaves of the tree will do; a time for new beginnings. It always appears impossible until it's done; be kind to you, the type of kindness that the blind can see and the deaf can hear; beating yourself up will not change what is happening; kindness definitely will.

One of the things I crave for is some normality in my life; to have a conversation that does not involve cancer, to get back to my daily routine. I find negativity surrounding cancer" The Big C" or "The C word, the word we are not allowed to say" is absolute nonsense; it feels as I am to blame for my situation; I am some sort of leper or freak, I am so fragile that I cannot cope.

Most of the problems that occur in relationships are caused by what is not being said, rather than what is said. Non-communication is simply another way of us all holding back from the real situation and how everyone is feeling; how everyone is coping. Not communicating openly and honestly can cause mistrust or come across as being false or insincere; it is like asking a Turkey if they are looking forward to Christmas or offering a person who is drowning a glass of water; what is the point? What are you trying to achieve? Please speak normally and openly; keep it positive and progressive; this really helps me have some normality; and I am certain it will benefit you as well.

I suppose having cancer nothing will ever be normal again; even if cured, it will still have an effect on my life in some way; will it come back? What life changes will I have to make? I understand that I will need to reset my life style, diet, to live as close to a normal life as possible; life does not come with a remote control, so to make these changes, I will have to get off my bottom and implement them, not waiting on others to do them for me. Again it means being positive and pro-active as opposed to sitting around feeling sorry for oneself. Caner is a family disease; I may be the one who has it; however the rest of my family suffers; I believe by being positive, involved in my own care and being seen to be getting on with life, this helps reduce that burden on them. If you step back and think about it; it is only the right thing to do anyway.

Last night Sam, my youngest daughter boyfriend was over for dinner; as I mentioned earlier my hair has started to fall out. He asked me if I was going to do Movember (growing a moustache to raise funds for male cancer); after ribbing him for being insensitive and taking the mickey out of me; I replied "No not this time, I may do Baldecember this year instead as a more viable alternative".

It is five days since I have had my autoinfusion pump removed; I am experiencing quite sharp pains in my lower chest/ oesophagus. The pains are quite acute, frequent and last for about 30 seconds; these have been present now for about 3 days. When on chemotherapy, any sign of chest pain needs addressing fairly promptly as it can come from a number of causes; some of these causes can be life threatening; Stroke, Angina, Blood Clots, Vasospasms for example; chemotherapy can cause my blood to thicken and inflame blood vessels and nerve endings making them very sensitive. When receiving chemotherapy you are more at risk from blood clots as you blood tends to congeal; trying to stay active can reduce this, as long as it is balanced up with rest. Immobilising oneself completely will throw up more complications; even when you do not feel like it, try gently moving about to keep the circulation flowing around the body. After speaking to St. James Hospital about my chest pains, I was told to go to A&E Immediately to be examined as chest pain raises a red flag for them. I went to Harrogate Hospital as this is my closest Hospital; here I was dealt with very rapidly, no waiting and kept away from the general public as being on chemotherapy, you are classed as high risk of infections. I had a number of tests, ECG, Blood Counts, give medication intravenously to reduce the spasms, physical examination. Whilst this was going ahead, the Oncologist Consultant was in contact with St James Hospital and had access to my medical notes; it is really comforting that they readily share information. After a couple of hours, the Oncologist Consultant came down to A&E to see me with the GI nurses. He explained that everything was normal from my ECG, Bloods and other medical examinations and that he would prescribe me some medication to reduce the spasms in my chest. He also explained that the pain I was experiencing was the chemotherapy attacking the tumour trying to break it down as it is designed to do. It was really nice that he took time out of his busy schedule to come down and chat to me and to reassure me that all was ok and given a further explanation of what was happening; he was hopeful after my third cycle of chemotherapy, I should be more or less pain free. After this I was discharged with some medication and went home; the attention and professionalism I received at Harrogate Hospital was outstanding.

We touched on how stress and anxiety has an effect on your body; Strokes, angina and vasospasms can be exaggerated by stress and anxiety. It is very difficult when caught in a situation like this; again is the unknown of what is happening to you. The importance of remaining calm at all times and removing the negativity from the situation is vital; it can be very unhelpful to your health both short and long term if you do not, staying calm helps you think clearly, make informed decisions to resolve the situation timely and effectively; Please be careful.

As I progress through my treatment; I have become a sponge to soak up as much knowledge as I can from the professionals; this allows me some peace of mind as I have a better understanding of what is happening to me. Taking an active involvement in the management of my care helps me be more at ease with myself and able to respond to any changes accordingly.

I am now halfway through my chemotherapy treatment with cycle number 3 coming this week. I can attest that there is nothing more certain to break my spirit and resolve than facing pain and discomfort every hour of everyday. The constant hospital visits, the cocktails of medicines and chemotherapy being put into me daily and their side effects; my whole body aching; wanting some relief from being run down and abused. I must remain focused on my purpose for going through this and not giving up; not choosing comfort over reaching my finishing line. Don't give up even when overtaken by temporary defeat; rest but don't stop, keep on moving forward; it will eventually pass. Hopefully, one day you will tell your story of how you overcame what you are going through now, and it will become part of someone else's survival guide to get them through their tomorrow.

November 5th Pre Assessment for Chemotherapy Cycle Three

Today I attended my pre-assessment in preparation for cycle three of my chemotherapy treatment.

As with the other assessments, my weight and blood were taken to ensure my treatment is where it should be. From there I spoke with the Doctor about any side effects I had experienced from my last cycle so any adjustments can me made accordingly to my next chemotherapy treatment.

After taking into consideration my visit to A&E last week and my experience so far; the Doctor is happy to keep my treatment plan as the previous two cycles. Happy with the decision and speaking to the Doctor, I left the Hospital very positive and looking forward to getting on with my next cycle in two days' time.

The pre-assessment days are important and mainly just very routine; it just gives the medical teams time to adjust any treatment specifically to me and to monitor my progress through my journey. When I go to the hospital, the first thing I have each time is a blood test, this is two days before my next treatment cycle. It's important that the checks of my red blood cell count, white blood cell count are carried out before my next treatment. If my red blood cell count is too low, I may need a blood transfusion. If either my white blood cell count or my platelet count is too low, having more treatment could push them down to a level that isn't safe.

My blood tests also check how well my kidneys and liver are working. If they aren't working as well as they should, the chemotherapy may be giving me more side effects than anticipated. Some cancers produce chemicals (biomarkers) that can be found in the blood; the doctors take some blood to test for these markers. They can use it to see how well my treatment is working. After my blood has been taken, if everything's okay, I can go ahead with my treatment as planned.

If my blood counts are too low, then unfortunately my treatment will have to be delayed; I will get another appointment at a later date to come back and have another blood test; until they are happy with my blood counts, then treatment cannot proceed.

Noticing that my hair is starting to fall out now slightly quicker than previously; I also realised that my facial hair isn't growing, so no need to shave for a while. Just like the leaves that are falling from the trees now it is autumn, it will grow back signalling a new life is beginning. Apart from this, I feel quite well in myself and have actually put on 2 kg in weight which is also a good sign that chemotherapy is working; if it wasn't working, I would be losing weight quite quickly and finding it difficult to eat or drink.

November 7th Chemotherapy Cycle Three and following days

Today is the start of my third cycle of chemotherapy; FLOT the Mike Tyson of chemotherapy treatments; my body is ready the best it can be for what is coming its way.

I have followed the same routine as last time; taken my steroid tablets, anti-sickness tablets and changed to a soft food diet to help digestive system cope with constipation. I know that I am going to feel a bit rubbish for a number of days, however I believe it is working and I will be three quarters of the way through chemotherapy after this cycle.

St James Hospital is a massive Hospital in Leeds with its own purpose built specialist cancer wing dedicated to those suffering from cancer. One thing I still find difficult to get my head around is; as you leave the hospital car park to walk to the cancer wing, 100 yards or so across the hospital grounds; the amount of people outside who are cancer patients as the have drips attached to them, sitting in wheel chairs, in their pyjamas and gowns, outside in the cold damp weather, smoking. If people wish to smoke, that is fine that's their choice, it keep my taxes down as well; I just think that the medical staff inside are working their very best to help them, yet they are quite happy to keep nipping outside for a cigarette, puffing away on a cancer stick amongst the very prominent no smoking signs. Is this not counterproductive and defeating the object of what the hospital is trying to achieve for them? People need to take responsibility and accountability for their own health and not pass all that onto the medical teams. No amount of medicine will cure negativity; when you start being positive, you start to take care of yourself, you start to feel better, you start to look better, that change all starts with you. Cancer and being involved in your own care is not a topic to be avoided and one that needs to be faced head on with commitment; with a physical and mental life reset. I sincerely believe there is no excuse for not doing everything you possibly can to give you the best chance of beating this terrible disease. Maybe people may think my comments are like being told you're stupid by the village idiot; or is the habit of smoking far stronger than the desire to live?

The routine at the hospital was exactly the same; the nurses got to work on me straight away, busying themselves in their natural calm, efficient and professional manner as they have always done. Drips medication checked and cross checked and away we go.

As I mentioned previously, I love being surrounded by positive people and having the complete reverse view of negativity. Unfortunately today I had the most negative gentleman sitting next to me; I don't think he could complete a sentence without stating "he hates", wow this guy could give an aspirin a headache. He certainly would not make it as a motivational speaker. After a about an hour of being polite and nodding along hoping he would get bored; I started to lose the will to live. I said to him, "he needs to speak to one of the nurses if he has all these issues and maybe they can help him; I cannot help you and neither do I have the energy to listen to your moaning and groaning any longer" If he didn't like what I had said to him, he would have disliked immensely what I was actually thinking; my mind was like a devil on Tourette's; at least I engaged my brain before speaking. I cannot remember how many times I rolled my eyes around my head, I must have looked like a slot machine in a Las Vegas Casino, I was just desperate for peace and quiet. Now having a cocktail of steroids for breakfast; I believe there is something called Roid Rage, they can make you angry even at the slightest of irritations; wrongly of me, I could see this man is going to end up wearing his drip stand as a scarf if he continued. I told him "this conversation is going nowhere fast, it's like him revving his car engine without putting it in gear, he is making a lot of noise and not getting anywhere" When you continually moan about your problems to people, 80% of the people don't care you have them; I was in this group to start with; and the other 20% are glad you have them; after an hour I was firmly entrenched in this group. To get some peace and quiet, I pulled out some headphones from my bag and popped them in my ears; I left the plug end in my pocket, not connected to anything in the hope he thought I was listening to music. It worked; normal service resumes. I appreciate he may be suffering or not happy about things; however there are far better ways to deal with it than constantly moaning to someone who cannot help anyway. This is about taking responsibility and changing the situation, and that can only be done by thinking clearly and addressing the issues rather than burdening everyone else with his problem. Continually moaning just increases the problem each time, compounds it and makes you moan more the next time; it is not healthy and not conducive to your overall well-being. I am not judging this man, not at all; I have to concentrate on my own concerns and well-being without being burdened with someone else's concerns. As an example, he was "F-ing and blinding about having his sandwiches made with malted bread and not just brown bread; this went on for about 15 minutes; at the end of the day, he bought the sandwiches himself, so he knew what he was buying beforehand yet blames everyone else for his own mistake. Very wrong of me to say, but I wished the sandwich would take revenge on him for his painful moaning and choke him; nightmare. The situation that he finds himself in, blaming the world and everyone in it for his condition is not going to change by chance; it can only change by choice; and that choice to change lays fairly and squarely with him. In contrast to him, a lady who was in for her first chemotherapy cycle came in wearing a bright pink T.Shirt which she had made up, with the caption on; "My cure starts today 7/11/2019", what a wonderful, positive attitude and a great outlook on her treatment and her end goal. For me it is about looking at the situation I find myself in, how can I work with it rather than against it to make the best outcome possible with what I know; it will never be ideal; however it must be far better than blaming everyone else and expecting them to do it for you.

The rest of the day went according to plan; I was connect up to my autoinfusion pump and sent on my way. The pump appears to running to time this so hopefully it will be coming off when it is scheduled to, unlike last time which ran for a further 24 hours. No such luck, the pump ran for an extra 7 hours, so I had to wait until morning to have it removed, a slight inconvenience, at least all of the contents have been used and inside me.

Today at home our boiler has broken; not ideal time for it to happen, as the weather is starting to get really cold now, frosty mornings and evenings and colder days not really rising about 7 degrees during the day time. The engineer cannot fix or repair the boiler so a new one will have to be installed; unfortunately when the new hot water tank was installed, the engineers never connected up the immersion heater to a live switch; this means we cannot switch it on to access any hot water. The chemotherapy makes me very exposed to the cold; pins and needles shoot over my entire body as a side effect. Without the hot water and heating; this could lead to some further complications in my treatment; I cannot afford to get an infection through poor personal hygiene or poor hygiene standards within the house, all this can lead to a delay in my treatment and cause a huge set back in my recovery. If I pick up a cold; because my immune system is down, there is a distinct possibly it could lead to pneumonia; this is why the Oncologist continually tells me to keep wrapped up with hats and scarves. I tried explaining this to the engineer, which, unfortunately fell on deaf ears; all he was interested in was telling me what he could not do rather than what he could do; the boiler was working fine until he came out to service it. I am not an engineer, but I know the boiler could have been left in a safe working manner. This is the type of attitude I go on about, a defeatist attitude, unable to think outside of the box, not one ounce of creative or positive thinking. The whole negativity you are met with is quite breath taking and arrogant to put it mildly; I just can't abide by it. With any situation like this, we have to adapt to it and ensure we can make the best out of the situation, not throw in the towel at the first signs of trouble and giving up as an easy option. He could not slap a sticker on the boiler quick enough saying "do not use" and having it completely shut down and disconnected. One trait you will discover about people who are negative; they always have a problem for every solution"

A reason to be cheerful today is because it is our grandsons first birthday and the little party at our house will still go ahead for him. We have bought some portable heaters for different rooms to keep the house warm; we can boil water for washing and keeping things clean. It is not the best, but it works, it's a solution to ensure we do not let the little man down on his special occasion. Unlike the engineer and the sandwich man on the ward, it about trying to figure out what can be done rather than what cant; being in a negative frame stops a person from thinking clearly and unable to solve problems; they react to it rather than respond to it. "Rant over"

One of the chemotherapy drugs I am taking is Oxaliplatin, it is important to remember certain things about Oxaliplatin and its side effects. Whist receiving treatment with Oxaliplatin: avoid cold temperatures and cold objects; this is the drug that exposes me to the extremes of the cold.

Some precautions I can take are:

- Cover my skin, mouth and nose if I must go outside in cold temperatures.

- Do not drink cold drinks or use ice cubes in drinks.
- Do not put ice or ice packs on my body.
- Do not breathe deeply when exposed to cold air.
- Wear warm clothing in cold weather at all times. Cover my mouth and nose with a scarf to warm the air that goes to my lungs.
- Do not take things from the freezer or refrigerator without wearing gloves.
- Drink fluids warm or at room temperature.
- Be aware that metals are cold to touch especially in the winter. Wear gloves to touch cold objects including my house door, car door, or gate latches
- If my body gets cold, warm-up the affected part with warm water.
- Wash my hands often.
- Use an electric razor and soft toothbrush to minimize bleeding.
- Maintain good nutrition.

As you can see, exposure to cold temperatures can be serious and care needs to be taken at all times; hence the annoyance with the boiler engineer not grasping the seriousness of the situation. I had a cold shower this morning due to us not having hot water as the boiler is broken and did not bother to heat up a pan of water to bathe in. Speaking to my oncologist nurse about the exposure to the cold and the side effects of pins and needles; it was mentioned that having a cold shower could have sent my body into shock; it would have a similar affect as jumping into the open sea on a cold winter's day. It is definitely something that should not be done as it could potentially be fatal, especially when the body's immune system is down.

Apart from feeling tired and a bit nauseous, the discomfort of the side-affects are slightly easier to deal with this cycle; I believe a lot of it is down to working out what is working for me and what is not, diet, exercise, rest and so forth. Listening to my body and adjusting accordingly, making small changes here and there; I am not over analysing things and being consumed by it, just figuring things out as I go along. At his point in my treatment, I still believe that listening to the medical teams and blocking out everything else has helped me up to now with the side-effects of chemotherapy and my general well-being. Would I use the same approach again? Yes I would as it has served me well.

One thing I have just noticed is, my hair has slowly stopped falling out and I needed a shave this morning as my facial hair has grown slightly; is my body fighting back, being defiant from the suffering it has been through over the last few months? I think the hardest part for me in connection with side effects are probably:

- Exposure to cold temperatures
- Tiredness/Fatigue
- Nausea

These have been the ones I have had to manage more closely as they were having the biggest effect on me; I believe by managing these three, then the treatment would not be as harsh as it sometimes can be. It is coming up to five days after my last cycle of chemotherapy; generally I do start to feel slightly better at this stage.

I also believe that gentle exercise daily is very helpful, apart from getting me out of the house and helping with boredom, it keeps everything functioning correctly and keeps my appetite healthy.

I know I still have a very long way to go; I am already so far from where I used to be, and that achievement makes me feel so proud.

Next week I have cycle four; this can either be my half way point in the treatment or a third of the way through. I was scheduled to have four chemotherapy cycles and if the chemotherapy has been successful in shrinking the tumour, then I need surgery to remove it from my oesophagus. If it has not shrunk as it should, then I would need further cycle's chemotherapy after surgery.

"When being diagnosed with cancer all of a sudden I am propelled into a complex world of Medicine, Science, Specialists, Surgeons and Nurses. This world can be quite alien and confusing; vulnerability and a feeling of being overwhelmed consumed me. It is a world that I know very little about until I was exposed to it, placed in to the depths of a deadly disease and the medical teams who fight it on my behalf. If not careful, and I don't take proper care of my mind, cancer will sabotage it; cancer is the silent destroyer of body and minds". From my initial diagnosis, it was like being placed on a medical shuttle bus, the NHS Express; this efficient process kicks in immediately, everyone knows what is happening, operating like clockwork, knowing exactly what their role is in my treatment. I am now on my journey; appointments, treatments, hospital visits, the shuttle bus never stops, just drops me off for that days treatment and picks me up later and continues on its journey to my next drop off point. I am swept along in the process trying to understand each step as I go; it is a steep and fast learning curve getting my head around things and understanding what is happening to me.

The medical teams are there for me, from the start of my journey, during my journey and after my journey; they literally become a huge and important part of my life.

I have spent so much time at the hospital that I thought I was going to be invited to their staff Christmas party thinking I was one of their own.

I believe that I have changed since being diagnosed with cancer; I have become more appreciative of my family, friends and life in general. I have always loved my family and friends; having a deep appreciation for them, is something truly special; it is an understanding of why you love them unconditionally. I was walking the dogs earlier today through the country side and sat on a bench for a while; the stillness and quietness was beautiful; looking out across the fields where I could see farmers tending their livestock and crops. Their machinery may have changed over the years, but the principles remain the same, passed down through the generations; nurture and feed the land to produce crops to feed ourselves and their animals. I appreciate farming is a tough life, but a relatively simple life; maybe that is how I should have mine. Drop out of the fast lane and enjoy the simpler things in life, appreciate what is actually on our doorstep; appreciation is more important to me than success. Success is judge by others; appreciation is measured for me and my family through satisfaction.

I have also found myself opening up a lot more; I have always been a private person and said only what I wanted to say, kept it short and sweet. I great friend of mine for many years has always said to me that I'm still an enigma to him; not that there is anything wrong with that; it is just that I have never felt the need really opened up, until now. My wife, youngest daughter and I were chatting about anything and everything over dinner; my youngest daughter then quoted a line from my wedding speech for our eldest daughter's wedding which took place in September. I always wanted my eldest daughter to have a copy of my speech, which my wife inserted into the back of a photo album she had made for them. My speech had some fatherly advice for her as she goes ahead in married life; the speech was written in a way that she could refer to it if I was not around to help her if cancer got the better of me. For my other daughter to remember parts of it for her own use, I find heart-warming and happy that it had the impact I desired. The quote she remembered from the wedding speech "As you both lead your lives as a married couple, there will be days when things may not be so smooth; always keep in mind, it is you both against the problem, not you both against each other. There is a reason why a car has a big windscreen and a small rear view mirror. It is more important to see the big bright future ahead, than to focus on what has happened behind you". This is the same advice I used for myself with cancer, looking to a brighter future.

When I told my wife and daughter why my speech was written in the way it was and the reason for a copy to be given; they were quite shocked and never contemplated my thinking behind it. This opening up I have found beneficial for people to understand me, how my mind works and for me as well to express myself in a way I have never done before. I have always thought long and deep about things and to share my understandings or reasons behind my actions opens up a whole new world for others as well as me. One of the greatest acts of kindness a human can receive is to understand and to be understood.

November 19th Pre Assessment for Chemotherapy Cycle Four

Today I attended my pre-assessment in preparation for cycle four of my chemotherapy treatment, and fingers crossed my last cycle.

As with the other assessments, my weight and blood were taken to ensure my treatment is where it should be. From there I spoke with the Doctor about any side effects I had experienced from my last cycle so any adjustments can me made accordingly to my next chemotherapy treatment. When talking to the Doctor, she asked if I am managing to keep moving and taking gentle daily exercise. This is something that I do and quite regimented about; I take either two short walks or one slightly longer walk, depending on the weather, or how I am feeling. Today before my pre assessment I walked cross country for four miles; it is a route I would do regularly and roughly takes about 1 hour 2 minutes. It was a beautiful still, bright frosty morning so I did not want to waste the opportunity to get out there and enjoy it. Wrapped up with hat, scarf and gloves with two Jack Russell's I set off. Half way around the route I did start to feel tired, even walking at a slower pace than normal; I also noticed I started to have a feeling of nausea in my tummy at the same time. Anyway we carried on and eventually returned home in one piece, very tired and feeling quite sickly in the stomach. I mentioned this to the Doctor; she pointed out to me that with the treatment I am on, the more tired that I become, the more it increases the feeling of nausea and sickness. This is why the Doctors are very keen to keep the balance correct between gentle exercise and rest; not over exerting myself and keeping everything in balance

The Doctor is happy to keep my treatment plan as the previous three cycles and on the maximum dosage of chemotherapy. She also wished me good luck with my surgery which will take place between 4-6 weeks after my last chemotherapy cycle; she also mentioned that she never wants to see me in her office again; trust me the feeling is mutual; thank you for all your help and advice on my visit to you. This gave me confidence that the treatment so far is working; however, the final say will come down to Doctor U, the consultant oncologist once he has all the information and results to hand. For now, I am happy with the place I am in to date.

November 21st Chemotherapy Cycle Four and following days

Today is the normal routine, taking my steroids and anti-sickness tablets, changed to softer foods and drinking plenty of fluids. Hopefully this will be my last cycle of chemotherapy and then the PICC Lines can be removed in a few days' time; the main follow up is in a few weeks when I see Dr U the consultant Oncologist; who will let me know how the chemotherapy has gone thus far.

Just had my fourth and final pre-planned cycle of chemotherapy yesterday; all depends what the oncologist consultant says in December. I am still on a drip for another 48 hours and the PICC lines will remain in place until my review. It is easier to maintain them than reinserting new ones. The oncologists have really stepped up the ante on this one and going all guns blazing for the tumour, needless to say my body is being subjected to a continued onslaught of nausea and discomfort; this is worse than all the last three cycles combined. There definitely feels like there is a war zone taking place inside my body; as long as it's working that is all that counts at this stage. Interesting fact talking about a war raging inside of me; In July 1917, troops based in Belgium, reported a shimmering cloud around their feet and a strange peppery smell in the air. Within 24 hours they started to itch uncontrollably and developed horrific blisters and sores.

They'd been poisoned by mustard gas; one of the most deadly chemical weapons deployed in battle. Mustard gas can be absorbed through the skin, so gas masks were useless, even fully clothed soldiers weren't fully protected. Mustard gas went from the very real battleground of the WWI trenches into the frontline of cancer treatment; subsequent work launched the start of a new era of cancer treatment; in fact, nitrogen mustard derived chemotherapy is still used to treat some cancers today. The era of cancer chemotherapy began in the 1940s with the first use of nitrogen mustards and folic acid antagonist drugs. The targeted therapy revolution had arrived, many of the principles and limitations of chemotherapy discovered by the early researchers still apply today. By World War II; at least two dozen medical researchers transformed mustard agents into cancer treatments; derivatives of mustard gas; became a new form of cancer treatment.

Last night sleep was in short supply and my whole body was itching all over like I was lying in an ants nest, along with nausea, not the most pleasant of experiences. One of the drugs I am taking Oxaliplatin does affect my nervous system, most commonly affected are in my hands and feet; however it can affect the entire body. This type of nerve damage is called peripheral neuropathy. As an example of this; at one stage I thought I was getting Bell's palsy as one side of my face became completely numb and I had no control over the muscles or movement in my face; everything in my face and mouth felt tight and drawn back to one side; be prepared for strange things to happen at random with chemotherapy.

I was out taking a little walk with the dogs earlier and being sensitive to cold temperatures I wear a hat, scarf and gloves all the time whilst out and about. My nose started to run so a quick sniff should solves the problem; wow, the pain up my nostrils and sinuses around my eye sockets was excruciating. That was completely unexpected, it had a feeling of being smashed across the bridge of my nose with a cricket bat; although it only last about five minutes, it was a very painful five minutes. This chemotherapy does weird and unimaginable things to the body, especially in very high doses. At least after the 1st night I can understand how the effects are playing out and try and respond accordingly through medication, rest and diet. Fingers crossed there is no more cycles after this one. Next time I will not be lazy and reach for the tissue in my pocket to wipe my nose rather than sniffing.

When I finished my cancer treatment and being given the all clear from this disease; you can ring a bell as you leave the ward to announce to everyone that you have beaten cancer. Generally other people in the vicinity will applaud and cheer for me, happy I am cancer free. I chose not to ring the bell; it does not work for me on a few different levels. Even though it does not work for me, I have absolutely no objections to other people ringing the bell; that's their choice and right to do so. The reasons for me not ringing the bell are important for two different reasons.

1 personal

2. Mindfulness of others

Personal
- When I had cancer I did not broadcast it to the world and kept it to close family and friends only; so I'm not going to broadcast my situation now to the world.
- From the beginning I have always said I will never be a victim to cancer, so there are no winners or losers here; just the outcome I expected.

- This time I am cancer free, am I tempting fate, I've had it once, there is every possibility I could get it again.

Mindfulness of others
- My youngest daughters very close friend and family lost their mum to cancer, a devastating impact on them. I have an image of the family, mum, dad, sister's sitting there by the bell, knowing that their mum will never get the chance to ring it. Knowing that cancer is taking their mum and wife away from them. Ringing the bell on my part is like gloating, rubbing salt into their already painful wounds.
- What about everyone else in the same situation that, are not going to survive, on palliative care only, sitting there without hope. I am sure they are pleased for the ones ringing the bell; however, how does it make them feel deep down?
  They will question why them? What have they done wrong not to survive? Why haven't the medical team saved them? Why has god been cruel to them? They will blame

themselves for their illnesses, something they are not responsible for. It will further increase their stress and anxiety, adding more pressure on a situation that is already desperate for them and their families.

- I could not allow myself to bring more misery to another family who are suffering enough in the knowledge they may not survive. So ringing the bell for my own personal happiness is not as important as having empathy with others not so lucky.
I will share my happiness in the privacy of my own home, in respect of those who will not be able to share their happiness with their loved ones. I would rather take a moment and think about them and hope that somewhere, someday they can find happiness again; hopefully a cure can be found soon for this disease that is so destructive and touches all of our lives.

I want people to be mindful of my own situation and what they say to me; I truly believe we should also be mindful towards everyone, no matter what their situation is. As previously stated, every action or inaction, everything we say or don't say carries a consequence. Please have self-awareness about those consequences of the well-meaning things you do or say, it can put the other persons mind into overdrive and a downward spiral, often into free fall.

Although I'm feeling like death warmed up for a while during this fourth cycle, so pleased this part is ending; it's better than just death I guess. It still amazes me how much punishment the body can take and keeps on going no matter what the discomfort levels it has. My results should be in 5/12/19 then on to the surgeon if all is well in early January to have the tumour removed. Hopefully he has a large family and can practice his knife skills on carving the turkey before being let loose on me. As long as he does not mistake me for the Christmas pudding and set me a light for the table centre piece.

Please continue to support people like me, we desperately need it; we just need it in the right form that helps us through our treatment and along our journey. Without your help, it would certainly be a journey that is a lot tougher to make; don't walk in front of me to protect me, don't walk behind me to push me along, walk beside me and share the journey I am on.

With cancer statistics as high as they are, the reality of you helping many other cancer patients, whether they be family or friends, are very high; the same principle will apply to them. Cancer casts long and dark shadows across all family members when one of their loved ones are suffering; when you reach out with kindness to support them in their time of need, be very mindful of their plight.

Your kindness, unconditional love and support are needed all the time; we just ask that all that effort is delivered in a way that is personalised, as every person's journey is different, and in a way that inspires us to continue. True friendship and kindness in our modern society is sometimes hard to come by; I am truly blessed to have it in abundance from my family, friends and the medical teams- thank you all, without you being there, who knows if a different outcome may of occurred. I am not there yet; however, through your help and support, I am one step closer to my finish line than I was yesterday.

My auto infusion pump has ran to time and the district nurse has been out to disconnect it and changing the dressing; it feels good to have it off as it makes it a lot easier to do simple tasks without having to carry it around with you and a trailing tube connected to your arm from it. For me, it just gives me a boost when it is disconnect, not sure exactly why, it just makes me feel better in myself. I am feeling slightly better today, probably more tiredness than anything, with a bit of constipation thrown in for good measure; saying that, things can change quite quickly for me over the first week of treatment. One moment I can feel okay, the next I could be at rock bottom, feeling as rough as houses; it is a matter of taking the good bits whilst they are available. The constipation from last night was not good; I sat on my bed from midnight to about 5.30 am without sleeping; because I can become so bloated from it, it can push the diaphragm upwards towards my chest making it difficult to breathe from the pressure. Hopefully today I can sort this out and feel more comfortable and have a sleep later on in the day.

This is something I really struggle to get my head around whilst sitting in the chair at St James Hospital having my chemotherapy. Smoking and cancer are related; smoking is the biggest cause of cancer anywhere in the world; the good news is; it is the biggest preventable cause of cancer in the world; if you stop smoking. The link between smoking and cancer is very clear. It causes at least 15 different types of cancer. Smoking causes around 7 in 10 lung cancer cases in the UK, which is also the most common cause of cancer death. Yet the guy sitting next to me, a 47 year old who had previously had cancer four years earlier, went out every hour on the hour, with his drip for a cigarette. It is certainly up to him what he does, surely logic or a dose of reality should have kicked in after first cancer four years earlier. The other unfortunate thing about him continually nipping out for a cigarette; you end up sitting next to someone who stinks like an ash tray for the next 6 hours or so; not very pleasant at all. I know it is his life and body to do with it a he wishes; with someone trying to save him on one side of the equation and himself appearing not caring on the other, does not make sense, the cost involved in his care and medication; someone in desperate need of help could benefit far more from treatment than him. "Is he really serious about his health"? There is a question that we should ask ourselves, "Am I willing to give up the things that are making me sick"

Thinking about his situation and the situation I find myself in has got my mind in overdrive. When a loved one falls ill, and a member of the family is faced with a critical condition; it highlights just how vulnerable we as humans are underneath it all; it can force us face some fundamental truths in life that we have maybe avoided or not dared to face up to along the way. The foundation of our human relationships and emotional state can be tested to the full; our ability to understand what is and isn't important to our core values and beliefs, what we will and won't do when faced with a crisis; and how different our own actions will differ from those around us. Through life we very rarely discuss our own vulnerabilities and insecurities; maybe it is a sign of weakness? When you find yourself in a situation like cancer, those emotions can come flooding to the surface and because we have never dealt with them in the past, they are quite alien to us, not knowing exactly how we are going to respond to it. This is what happened when I was sitting in the recovery ward after my endoscopy; these emotions surfaced and I honestly believe we do not know how we will respond until we are face to face with our fears. We can say "I will do this or that", I am not convinced as our emotions can be very powerful and override any thought process we have if we are not careful. A fake smile may hide a thousand tears; it won't though stem the flow. When faced with a situation like this, we have to be honest with ourselves and honest with others; bottling feelings up does not help in the long run; be open and keep the mind running clearly and freely. The communication channels need to be kept open with honesty; this way everyone can be understood and others can understand. Only then, can face the challenges that lay ahead; as one and with one united objective, to beat cancer and get through this with a successful outcome.

Sure there will be times when it feels life has me pinned up against the wall, everybody experiences that. It comes down to how I think about the situation, how I feel about it and how I respond to it.

The more I think in a negative frame of mind and feed the feelings the more I will feel low, resulting in negative behaviour of worthlessness, hopelessness and helplessness. If that spiral continues and gets stronger; then it becomes a habit, a process I have learned as a coping mechanism. So, if it started with a negative thought, wouldn't the best cure be changing my thought process to a more positive frame of mind and eventually change my feelings and behaviour to one that enhances me to live a happier and fulfilling life. So if it is a learned behaviour, a habit, it is possible to unlearn it and replace it with a habit that is more useful to me.

I am into my third day after having the auto infusion pump removed; I have to say this is the worse I have felt after any of my previous chemotherapy cycles. I haven't slept properly for this period, so feel quite exhausted at this moment in time. I have had bad headaches, my teeth have ached, feeling of nausea and like on cycle two, I can feel the chemotherapy attacking the tumour in my oesophagus; there is not the spasms like last time, just a burning sensation in the area of the tumour. Whilst this is a good sign, it does not feel pleasant at the time it is happening. I am hoping that this will wear off in a couple of days if it follows the same pattern as the last three cycles; however, nothing appears as it seems with my chemotherapy and it throws out new side affects all the time.

Having had my fourth planned cycle of chemotherapy; I do believe there is a lot to be said for a person's mental approach to illness and their own well-being. For me, I do think it plays a large part in my recovery and how it impacts on other people around me; I can quite easily talk myself into a negative state of mind that can spiral out of control or I can talk myself into a positive, healthy state of mind that can keep moving me forward. It really is about how I am focusing my mind. There is a saying "seeing is believing" I prefer to turn that on its head and rephrase it to "If I believe it, I will see it" and that is how I have had the focus of my mind since being diagnosed with cancer; if I believe I will get better, then I will see the positive results. Whoever or whatever has control of the mind, will generally win in the end. My body eaves drops on all my thoughts and words, it will then respond accordingly to what it has heard; as Henry Ford mentioned " If you believe you can or if you believe you can't; you are right".

Day five after my auto infusion pump was removed and I am starting to feel slightly better; still tired, but the nausea and chest pains are easing off. This seems to be the pattern from the previous three cycles and I have to admit, it is nice to feel a bit more human and comfortable; hopefully it stays this way until surgery. The one thing I notice above all since having chemotherapy is the tiredness; things I would normally do like walking the dogs, gardening, washing the car, work; these I find now are quite tiring to do, normally I would just blast through them and carry with my day. At this moment in time; I do feel the effects of tiredness even after gentle exercise; I have slowed right down from dashing around at 100mph; this will hopefully correct itself over the coming months. This is probably the hardest and most frustrating part of the whole treatment I have to deal with; trying to accept that I cannot do what I could do previously without feeling completely shattered. Everyday simple tasks end up being a huge chore; fatigue affects not only the body, it also affects the mind and how I am feeling; it is draining and leaves you exhausted. Worrying about cancer and letting it consume every minute of my day will also take its toll on me; I mentioned previously that cancer is like the school bully and needs attention to thrive; if I continually think about it and worry about it, it will punish me more than it does now. I've accepted cancer is there; the medical teams are fighting the battle for me and the side effects from chemotherapy are a constant reminder I have it; there is no need for me to pile more pressure on myself. If I ignore it and continue as normal as possible; like the school bully, it just becomes a minor irritation, a non-entity, starved of attention, it loses its power and control, unable to bask in its own self-imposed egotistical status.

I am nine days in after receiving my latest cycle of chemotherapy; it feels as though my body is returning to a more normal state; most of the pain, discomfort and nausea have virtually gone and I am not taking any medication at all at this moment in time. I know the chemotherapy is still swirling around my body; it is nice though not to be putting further medicine inside of me, allowing my body to function as it should without the aid of help.

The Hospital (LGI) phoned this morning; I have a CAT scan on the morning of the 5th December and then on to see the Consultant Oncologist the same afternoon. I am not sure if the results of the scan will be ready for the consultant in such a short period of time; hopefully they will be able to get them through at very short notice. If they are able to do this; then I will have a fuller picture of where I stand since starting chemotherapy and the extent as to how much it has worked.

In myself I believe it has worked, to what degree I obviously do not know and that can only be revealed from the scan. I am eating better, food is not getting stuck on a regular basis in my oesophagus, my weight has stabilised and I am feeling pretty happy within myself. Having put my body through chemotherapy and enduring its side effects; it better have done what it was intended to do, either stop the tumour growing and/or shrinking it. I am a firm believer that my state of mind contributes to my overall well-being; it cannot keep at bay all illnesses, like now with me having cancer; however it can certainly reduce the causes of some illnesses through removing stress, anxiety, depression and any negative impacts on the body. Conditions like stress, anxiety and depression are precursors to becoming ill and putting me at a greater risk to all kinds of diseases; cancer, diabetes for example. For me, having cancer now, this is the first time I have ever taken any time off work through any sort of illness; that's not to say I haven't been ill; it is how I have actually dealt with that illness. I am generally not a person who gets ill very often and that's because I have a very positive outlook on life and keep my mind healthy at all times. If I think about the amount of energy my body has used to get me to through chemotherapy, to where I am today; it is huge, delving into its reserves constantly to keep me going. This same amount of energy will be required to get me through my up and coming surgery and recovery from it. Now imagine the amount of energy and strength it takes to pull oneself out of a very dark place mentally; it is colossal, I really don't think people understand the amount of effort that this actually takes. Combine that with the energy needed to get through chemotherapy; or any illness, the bodies energy levels will be depleted, running on fumes; recovery therefore will be a lot harder and a lot longer. Keeping a healthy state of mind, has a very positive impact on the body and keeps those energy levels up to fight disease and not using them up to fight internally against myself. You give life to anything you give energy to.

"The strength of mind is always more powerful than the strength of body"

This statement is very important; if I think in a positive way, then my body will respond accordingly in a positive way. If I think in a negative way, my body will also respond accordingly, in a negative way. My body will always respond to how I think.

"Please stay away from negative people; they complain about everything and appreciate absolutely nothing" This is about you and not them.

It's a state of Mind

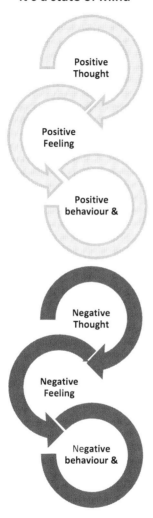

Positive Thought

Positive Feeling

Positive behaviour &

Negative Thought

Negative Feeling

Negative behaviour &

December 5th Chemotherapy cycles finished, visit to see Dr U the Oncologist Consultant. & CT Scan at the LGI

A CT scan is special X-ray tests that produce cross-sectional images of the body using X-rays and a computer. This will be used to determine how effective the four cycles of chemotherapy have been; it can also pin point which vessels are supplying the tumour with the blood supply it needs to grow. The scan results will be available for the Surgeon Mr S to work out the best way forward and most effective way to perform the operation. The operation to be performed; will be to cut out the remaining tumour and the affective part of the oesophagus.

I had the CT scan this morning, unfortunately and understandably the results will not be ready for a week; this means that my anticipated appointment this afternoon with Doctor U the Consultant has been pushed back by a week. It is disappointing as this is first of the dates or markers on my journey that was pencilled in and very important for me. The reason for this rearranged appointment is to allow him to get the results of the CT scan so he has a complete picture of how well the chemotherapy has worked and how we are going to proceed from here going forward. This can only happen once the radiologist has had enough reasonable time to interpret the results from my scan.

The CT scan was routine and nothing untoward; the only place they could insert the cannula was in my left index finger, right on the top knuckle. This was the only vein they could get blood from on the day; I must admit it was quite painful having it in my finger as it very close to the bone.

The CT scan results will be sent over to Doctor U as soon as they have been analysed and interpreted; although the appointment has been pushed back, it will not change the outcome of the results; it just means I have to be patient and wait a little longer to find out.

"I do believe I have won this battle, not the war yet though; that victory is still to come".

It has been two weeks now since I had my last chemotherapy cycle; it feels good not to be taking any form of medicine and allowing the body to recover and deal with it in its own way. I feel really good; I still suffer from fatigue; however the pain and discomfort associated with chemotherapy has virtually gone.

I received the date for my rearrange appointment with Dr U the consultant Oncologist; this is now a week away on 12th December.

November 12th Results of the chemotherapy treatment

Well today has finally arrived, my first major marker in my recovery programme; the day of my results from the chemotherapy treatment. From how my body feels now from where it came from, I am expecting positive results from my meeting. I always believed that this ugly part of my story which I am living through right now; would become one of the most positive parts of my life in how to deal with adversity; an extremely profound period in my life.

The scan results revealed that the chemotherapy has worked; shrunk the tumour and stabilised it enough to perform surgery. This means I will now move to the next phase of my treatment; surgery in early January. Although I understand what the surgery entails, I have to meet the surgeon again to find out exactly how he plans to perform surgery now he has the full results. Mr S has a number of options open to him and will meet with the medical teams first and then myself to discuss his thoughts and preferred option.

All in all, a positive result today and I am a happy man; 50% of the way through my journey and I have been discharged from the oncology department. I believe that the next 50% (surgery) is really tough, or as the surgeon said it, "brutal". I will adopt the same approach of being mentally strong as I was with the chemotherapy, it served me well then and it will do the same now. I coached, mentored and counselled myself through that period, using the great support from family and friends to prop myself up on. I will again only base my decisions on the advice of those who will share the consequences of this disease I have. I will remain practical and optimistic at all times; being positive also attracts the people you come into contact with to respond positively. The teams give information to you straight as it is, rather than dampening it down as they know you can take it. Being positive makes everyone's life easier; they don't have to tread on egg shells around you, worried that they can upset you with a slip of the tongue. Most importantly, my body responds accordingly, my mind stays focused and uncluttered, which can only aid my recovery.

So for now I will enjoy Christmas before I refocus my mind on the surgery and prepare myself mentally for it.

Until then, using the words of the chorus from the famous Christmas song by Slade;

> "So here it is, Merry Xmas
> everybody's having fun
> Look to the future now
> it's only just begun"

I guess those words carry a more important message for me now.

"Merry Christmas everyone"

Summary for Stage one of my treatment

- Accept you have cancer; denying it or not accepting it does not change the situation. Accepting it does.
- Have an open mind, accept all the facts and information that your medical teams give you.
- Clear your mind from external noises and listen to the people who share the consequences with you
- Face cancer head on and do not be afraid of it.
- Create a positive mind set and maintain it at all time
- Focus on where you are now and what you want; not where you are now and what you don't want.
- Accept chemotherapy is going to be uncomfortable and some days will be rough. The discomfort is only temporary.
- Set markers or goals to achieve along your way; and celebrate each victory, no matter how small.
- Find out what works for you and what doesn't during chemotherapy; diet,

exercise; rest, what you are capable of; adjust as necessary to reduce the discomfort.

- Trust in the medical teams and your own body to fight the battle for you.
- Each day is one day closer to your finish line; irrespective how long that journey is. You are one day closer than you were yesterday.
- Be honest with yourself and with others; share information
- Make sure your loved ones are in a good place at all times.
- Believe you can do this, even on those bad days when everything appears impossible, never give up ever. It's a state of mind and you control that state.

I genuinely believe 100% that if I can get three things right before chemotherapy treatment starts and maintaining it throughout my treatment; I will have a far greater chance of being cancer free and reduce my recovery time. Although I have mentioned getting these three parts right before my treatment starts; it should be a way of life anyway; as it can only benefit me each and every day to live a healthier life. Having the right mind set is a choice; a life style choice and everything I do, stems from my thoughts and the way I think about things. Having a negative thought process will slow down my recovery time and increase anxiety and frustrations.

1. Having a healthy state of mind: this will ensure that I can make the correct decisions and respond accordingly to my treatment. It will also make sure that the following two parts happen; without this positive mental approach, all else fails. I have counselled and mentored myself through this; find a professional person to help you create the mind-set essential to recovery and health, it all starts with the

mind; the mind determines everything else for the body.

2. To get as fit as possible: this will ensure my body can take the treatment and surgery. It will help to keep my body in a healthy state through its punishing regime of chemotherapy and surgery, giving it the best chance to fend off infections, pain and discomfort. It will have more of the necessary resources to respond to treatment and reduce some medication intake. I don't need to be a super fit athlete or join a gym, just gradually improving my level by walking, being active and doing; rather than being a couch potato.

3. Having the correct nutrition and diet: this makes sure my body is getting the correct food and nutrients it needs and not what it just wants to have. It will help repair itself, maintain a healthy weight and provide the strength it needs to keep moving forward. There are seven major classes of nutrients; carbohydrates, fats,

fibre, minerals, proteins, vitamins and water. Please discuss with your nutritionist and follow their guidelines. It does make a difference as with the other two parts. Ask the question "do I live to eat or do I eat to live"?

All three parts are completely dependent to each other and each individual part needs the other two parts to perform and maintain me at a level to increase my survival chances and recovery. The healthy mind-set is the engine of the three, the driving force of the formula. Lose one of the three parts or unbalance the healthy mind-set; and I have just stacked the odds in favour of the cancer.

Get all three parts fully aligned and working together as one; I will take the same situation like cancer, which many people have complained about and I will win.

Three Part Formula for Success

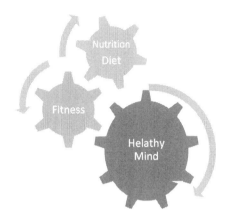

I knew that I would have to make changes to my lifestyle after my treatment; it is fairly obvious to me that those changes need to benefit me both in the short term and long term. Why wouldn't I make those choices based around the three part formula? For me they are the heart-beat of a healthy life style, the key drivers and an obvious choice. Not following them or basing my lifestyle changes around them, can only be counterproductive and makes a mockery of what I have just been through over the past year. "It does not make sense at all, no matter how you try and dress it up"

December 20th Harrogate A&E

Earlier on in the week I woke up about 1.30 am in extreme discomfort; the pain in my chest and abdomen was literally excruciating. At first I thought it maybe a touch of food poisoning or the norovirus which does the rounds every year at this time. I vomited eight times in total during the early hours of the morning; this did relieve some of the pain in my upper body, but not the abdomen area. For the rest of the day I did not eat a thing and just lay on the bed feeling really poorly, unable to do anything, concentrate on anything; I just want to lay there in silence.

On the Tuesday morning after a very rough night, diarrhoea started which in a way I was happy about, happily getting this bug out of me by passing through the system. I was able to eat light food, like soup, which fortunately stayed down and at least lined my tummy. My stomach and lower abdomen area was very tender to the touch, any form of pressure on it really hurt and gave me a feeling of nausea. The worst area was around the top right hand part of my upper abdomen, just below the diaphragm and in the area of the liver. This pain increased to such a level, I was unable to walk, only shuffle, unable to get in and out of a chair unaided, get on and off my bed; any form of pressure on my core was exceptionally painful and debilitating; even my breathing was shallow.

I decided to go to the hospital for two reasons; I did not want any complications to delay surgery in January to my oesophagus, and secondly, I needed to find out what was happening to me at this moment in time. After a couple of hours or so in A&E, carrying out a series of tests, X-rays, ECG, Bloods and so forth, the Doctor said they were waiting for an abdominal surgeon to come and examine me. The surgeon arrived and after a couple of minutes of questioning, a brief examination of my stomach; he said that I will be admitted into hospital as they need to treat and sort out my gallbladder which was infected, inflamed and swollen. This was a possible side effect from the chemotherapy, were my immune system being completely low, the gallbladder is unable to protect the body at this moment in time by moving through waste from the liver. I was quickly hooked up to a drip of antibiotics whilst a bed was found and an ultra sound scan arranged for me. Once a bed was found, I was on a strict course on antibiotics given intravenously for a couple of days in the hope to reverse the damage on the gallbladder; along with this, plenty of rest was needed.

I cannot believe that such a small organ in the body can cause pain so excruciating and debilitating; the good thing to come out of this is," at least it was the chemotherapy causing the problem and not the cancer itself"

When the Doctors admitted me to the ward and placed me on a drip they asked me, probably a routine question; however when I been through months of pain, discomfort, fatigue, injections, hospital visits, nausea, diarrhoea, chemotherapy; the mental pressure and physical pain is massive and exhausting. I know that surgery is only a few weeks away and the whole scenario is going to repeat itself again for the next few months; and then I am are asked this question "if for any reason due to your condition; you need to be resuscitated, do you want us to perform the resuscitation or not".

Think of all the months of pain I have gone through and still have to come and I am asked a question " do you want to live or die" whilst doubled up in complete agony both physically and mentally exhausted. Is the answer as easy as you think? This question is very challenging; especially when I am tired of being tired, and pain appears to be my closest friend. However the question is answered; the doctors are obliged to carry out your request; the answer will determine my fate. It is essential that I am looking after my mind; as I never know what is around the corner and how I am going to respond to the given situation; it literally could be life or death. Even with a strong mind; a momentary lapse of determination, being temporarily over taken with pain; can change that answer from three letters to two.

I have finally been discharged from hospital to finish my recovery at home; I can now take anti-biotic medication orally so they were happy to let me go. I have made progress, slowly, but responding well to the treatment I have received from the hospital; hopefully I can now enjoy Christmas and relax before the next challenge in January.

The date of my surgery has finally been confirmed; 09/01/2020- this is the date my New

Year starts and rid my body of this unwelcome guest who has been lurking there for the past year. My surgeon has changed to Mr D; who by all accounts is an extremely talented surgeon, and I am assured that my health is in very, very capable hands. This hopefully will be my final push to the finish line; then I can carry on with life as normal, pain free and redirecting my energies to the things I wish to pursue, rather than just recovering.

When cancer hits you, it hits you very hard; a sucker punch that takes the wind out of my sails. The one thing it does not like, is hitting it back; just like the school bully, it is not as tough as it thinks it is. There is only one way to deal with cancer, and that is to deal with it; no excuses, no alternatives, no denials, face it head on and deal with it.

During the treatment, I will have set backs and days that haven't gone so well; it is not about how many setbacks or falls I have along the way; it is more important about how many times I get up and carry on going. Cancer has knocked me down a few times; it showed me things I never wanted to see. I have experienced sadness and a sense of failure, but one thing for sure, I always got back up. When I do have these setbacks and going through a rough time; just sit with me, no preaching, no advice, no comparing; just be there. It is amazing sometimes just how much the silence can be so comforting and helpful; it can bring an inner peace and strength through calmness; a quieting of the mind. Enjoying the silence and just being is a very powerful tool and part of the healing process for the body and mind.

This week is the week for my operation; it was a great psychological boost for me today, completing a walk I usually do in the same time as I would normally do it in before chemotherapy started; generally it has been taking me 50 minutes longer than normal. This tells me the body is recovering well and getting back to a level of strength and fitness I need to take on surgery. Getting back to this level will certainly boost my recovery and general well-being; hopefully it will get me on my feet sooner and back home to get on with life. Any little advantages gained to help me along the way are just as important as the larger ones;

everything adds to my recovery no matter how large or how small.

January 7th Meet Mr D (Surgeon) & Pre Assessment for surgery

Today I have just had met the surgeon Mr D who is going to perform my operation. This was quite straight forward were he went through exactly how he intends to carry out the surgery (keyhole surgery), what is involved and what I should expect when I awake from surgery and the recovery period that lays ahead for me. This was pretty straight forward; I asked a few questions so I could fully understand the whole procedure pre-operative and post-operative, this for me removed any doubt, uncertainty and left me with a clear view of the challenges that lay ahead for me.

Mr D said it will be about a 10 hour operation, followed by 4 days in a High dependency unit and then up to 12 days on a normal ward. Mr D will do keyhole surgery (10 entry points) and one larger incision on my back. They will remove part of the stomach, lymph nodes and most of the oesophagus; whilst they are in there, they will also remove the damaged gallbladder. After surgery it is nil by mouth for about a week until the wound has healed around the oesophagus. The full recovery could be about 4/6 months; then learning to eat again and having the body getting used to its new lay out of the digestive system

From Mr D, I was then off for a pre assessment for the operation; however before that I was caught by the dietician who knew I was in the building. The dietician wanted to run through the foods I would be eating post –operative and to give me advice on my diet which will change quite dramatically after surgery, all the hints and tips I need about food, what to eat, what to avoid for the time being and so on. I have to admit this advice was invaluable during the very early stages of my recovery and put to rest any fears I had especially when food would not stay in my stomach or my weight was dropping too quickly.

The pre-assessment was just another formality, routine carrying out of my height, weight, blood pressure and a 12 page long questionnaire about my past health. I was helped by a nurse to fill this in as it quite long and laborious, albeit very important.

That was it really for the day; it was the final opportunities for the hospital to get me prepared for surgery and ensure they had all there information correct and up to date.

I think at this stage it was dawning on me that we are now at the real business end of the treatment; the cutting away of the scourge that has been living inside of me silently trying to destroy my body and mind. It was now time for us to part company, for good, its free tenancy has now come to an end and the scourge will be evicted from my body by the skills of Mr D and his dedicated team of professionals. This is the moment I have been waiting for since being diagnosed; having my body back and knowing that the cancer has now been removed. This thought removed any doubt, nervousness or concerns I may have had about surgery; I just wanted to get on with it now and get it over with and kill this tumour for good.

The surgery I will be having is a minimally invasive 2 stage Oesophagogastrectomy and a Cholecystectomy, this was to remove the damaged gallbladder which I had experienced just before Christmas. Mr D was combining two surgical operations into one; made a lot of sense to me

January 9th Day of the Surgery

The day has finally come around, and although it feels like an eternity, the whole procedure since being diagnosed to this point in time has been fairly rapid.

I have arrived at the hospital in plenty of time having fasted since early evening the previous night; it is still very quiet in the hospital (6.15am) and a lot of the place is in semi darkness. I head towards the admissions desk, only to be greeted by occupied beds in the corridors and checking in area. A nurse greeted me and took me to a side room and explained that A&E had had a seriously busy night and that there were no beds available as yet on the wards to move the patients to who had emergency surgery throughout the night.

More patients began to arrive who were booked in for surgery that day; obviously they walked into the same situation I had just witnessed and experienced the same over spill of patients in corridors on beds. A smile came across my face; with all the information that the hospital give you, they specifically asked people not to bring much personal stuff into the hospital as there is not enough storage space on the wards. People still manage to bring in huge suitcases as if they were off on holiday somewhere; you could see the nurses looking at the luggage thinking, if this was a flight you were catching, then you would be being charged extra for your bags being over the weight limit.

We were eventually moved to a different floor in the hospital where nurses and doctors where scurrying around trying to bring calm to a chaotic situation, brought on by the extremely busy night previously in A&E where a lot of the beds had been taken up. Sadly this situation led to most of the operations today being cancelled as there were no beds available. Fortunately my surgeon was able to carry out my operation as planned, and from a very selfish point of view, I was glad the cancellation of appointments was not mine today. Yes I did feel for the other people, but at this moment in time, it was more important for me to be seen. The surgery I will be having done is an oesophago-gastrectomy; Mr D will remove the top of my stomach and the part of the oesophagus containing cancer and then reattach them by stretching the stomach upwards. He will also remove my gallbladder at the same time. An operation to remove oesophageal cancer is major surgery and will take time to recover from it. During surgery Mr D will take out the lymph nodes from around my oesophagus and stomach, this helps to reduce the risk of cancer coming back; this is known as a lymphadenectomy. Mr D takes out lymph nodes in case they contain cancer cells that have spread from the main cancer in my oesophagus; it also helps the multi-disciplinary teams to decide if I will need chemotherapy after surgery.

I eventually ended up in theatre were the anaesthetists immediately began to set about me; I had an epidural inserted into my back and a cannula into the back of my right hand. I was given some oxygen and then administered the anaesthetic and told to enjoy my sleep by the gas man; that is the last thing I remember until I awoke on the recovery ward some twelve hours later.

When I came around on the recovery ward and gained my senses; I was definitely the human form of the Ker-Plunk game. Drains and tubes were poking out of my body, and a catheter thrown in for good measure to complete the set. It took a while for me to come around and to be honest, I did not feel any pain or knew what had happened or how the operation had gone; successful or not. The feeling of doing to many sit ups was all I could feel around my diaphragm; apart from that the epidural was obviously doing its jobs of pain relief.

After an hour or so I was transferred to the high dependency ward were I was hooked to lots of machines regulating oxygen and nutrients into my body. It was quite noisy on the unit, machines bleeping all the time and nurses busy moving around constantly checking my temperature and monitoring the statistics on the display screen above my head. I cannot say it was restful on the ward, but it was comforting to know that the care I was getting was exceptional and could not ask for more. The overriding feeling I had was of thirst, as it was nil by mouth, my mouth was very dry; I was given some small sponges on a stick to dip in water to be able to wipe the inside of my mouth. Whilst the moisture was welcome, it was not enough to try and quench my thirst; I believe at his stage the amount of fluid intake I was getting through the drip was increased, this did help a lot more and also helped me to pass more fluid through the catheter.

The next day after being washed and cleaned by the nurses, they managed to get me out of the bed and sitting up in a chair. Although I had drains and tubes everywhere, it was nice to be able to sit up right, get the lungs functioning again as they should. Being able to move also helps with the prevention of bed sores, these can be quite painful in themselves. Before the operation and trying to take control of my situation; I had discussed with my wife that for the first two days I did not want any visitors, I wanted to preserve all my energy for my recovery. After that only on visit per day until I left hospital for the same reason; I do find visits quite tiring and making conversation for the sake of it. For me I would rather use that time for deep relaxation and focus on my body healing from surgery. Since the start of my treatment I have had a tunnel vision, solely concentrated and focused on my recovery and this has not changed now even after the operation. That same level of focus and concentration of self-recovery is just as important now as it was in the beginning. Yes I can rely on medication and drugs to help me recover; I also have a responsibility to help myself and not just being reliant on others to do it for me. I have followed the advice of the medical teams from day one and continue to do so; I also know that there are things I can do to help myself also; for me is to get moving and continue with my deep relaxation and self-hypnosis.

When doing deep relaxation, my whole bodily functions slow right down, breathing, pulse and so on; this allows the body to be totally relaxed and repair itself naturally.

I believe that this illustration speaks volumes; we need to take responsibility for our own health and life styles in general, not just now but at all times. We should not be reliant on others and medicine to do the work for us; life does not come with a remote control; sometimes we have to get up and change things.

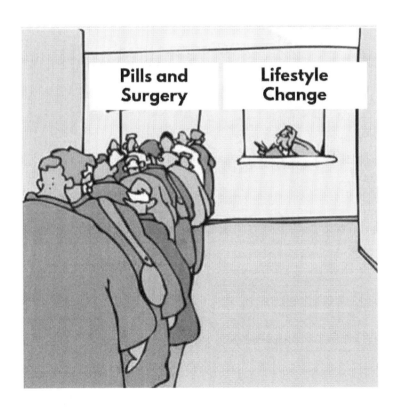

After three days of the normal routine of being monitored every four hours, I was eventually moved to a general ward in the cancer unit. This is a good sign, as for me, it says I am out of the immediate danger and making enough progress where I do not need the constant monitoring; I was also allowed to start sipping water, what a relief this was.

I had my first visit from family today which was lovely; I did pre warn them not to be shocked by the amount of tubes and drains sticking out of me; I felt it would benefit them and reduce the chances of being upset on seeing me for the first time since my operation.

It is quite nice on the ward; at least you get a chance to chat to fellow patients and the ability to move around more freely, especially after day four post operation. This is when a number of tubes were removed from my body which instantly makes me feel better. The only tubes left in were a cannula a PICC line in my neck and a chest drain; this was the thickness of my finger. The epidural had by now been switched off; I had no pain relief whatsoever being administered to me once the epidural was switched off, four days after surgery. To my surprise and to the surprise of the medical teams, I did not require any further pain relief; I honestly put this down to my deep relaxation, which I continue to do and to the focus on my recovery, all through a positive mind set. It was also nice to be able to go to the bathroom to wash, use the toilet and so on; getting my mobility and independence back.

During this time, I have had visits from the physiotherapists and dieticians; the physio has me walking around the full ward to start building up strength and to get the lungs working. At first it is difficult, but one foot in front of the other, each day my strength is building and soon I can do a few laps of the cancer wing. It is too easy to give up when discomfort strikes; it is having the determination to push through that discomfort and to keep moving.

So far my recovery is going exceptionally well, and probably slightly further ahead of where I should be at this stage; I am starting to eat sloppy foods now, only little amounts; however each mouth full builds up the much needed strength my body requires, especially since I am burning up energy by becoming active.

In hospital every day blends into the next with a much regimented routine day and night; the days and nights can be quite long. I chose those times to remain focused on my recovery and prevent the mind wandering in the endless boredom of being in hospital. Every day during the Doctors rounds, I wait for an update on my condition and wait for the magic words, "you can go home today". For me this sentence came on day 10; unfortunately I had picked up a slight infection which held back my discharge date.

Today is good news, day 10 since surgery; I can go home to continue my recovery in my own home with the support of my loving family. I have packed my bag, collected my medication and this is the thoughts I have on leaving the hospital:

On the 11th September 2019 cancer and I first walked into St. James Hospital. That scourge living inside of me. Today 20th January 2020 after numerous cycles of punishing chemotherapy and major surgery; my exhausted, battered and bruised body; minus a few parts, is walking back out of here; without the scourge. It's not an overly long walk to the car park, but after surgery of this nature, putting one foot in front of the other is very tough and tiring. I will walk out of St James Hospital slowly, step by step, unaided in a show of defiance to cancer, that no matter how hard it tried, that scourge hasn't broken me.

Who knows what the future holds, whether I have to make this journey again or not. For now it's a lovely feeling to return to my family and the wonderful people who have given me their support since day one, now its recovery time.

Each day now in my recovery I am getting stronger, becoming more mobile; it has been a long journey and still away to go. I honestly believe my recovery was enhanced through a positive mental approach from day one; having that unwavering focus on becoming better. I understand we are all different and our illness can affect us in different ways; however we can prevent it from affecting our minds. Remain focused and control what you can; every knock down, get back up and keep going.

For every time my mind went blank or with lost thoughts; if I inserted a blank page in this book each time that happened; most of it would consist of blank pages. It is those times when I needed to concentrate and remain stoic, and bring my mind back to reality so that it never once let me down.

My main focus now is diet, what works and what doesn't; this is just close monitoring of quantity, consistency of food, and what food remains inside me for long enough to have the nutrients absorbed from it.

Good luck with your journey, I hope some of my actions and thought process will help you along the way; even in those dark moments when you feel like someone has switched the light off at the end of the tunnel; keep travelling, you will get there eventually.

Remember the three essential ingredients of the formula

- A healthy Mind
- A healthy Diet
- Exercise

They will keep you in a good place and go a very long way to helping you defeat cancer and your recovery.

Conclusion

Finally I have crossed my finish line; chemotherapy and surgery have been successful and life is returning to some form of normality. I have to thank so many people who have helped me along the way, family, friends and the fantastic multi discipline medical teams across the NHS. One person who has been incredible over this time has been Fatima, my wife; she is truly one amazing person and without her constant help and care, this journey would have been a lot harder. Maybe that is why god did not take me this time, in the knowledge he has left me with one of his trusted angels to look after me for a while longer. "Fatima; if there is ever a time when we cannot be together, keep me in your heart and I will stay there forever; love you always".

To all the wonderful people in my life, this is my wish for you "May you always have happiness to keep you smiling and the belief that each day is a gift that we should make the most of"

Cancer is a horrible disease and I hope by supporting cancer research, they will find a cure sooner rather than later, with our support we can make this happen; we can provide the much needed resources for them to rid the earth of this disease that silently destroys our body and minds. Maintain a positive outlook at all times, do not fear cancer; face the challenge head on and control what you can control and let the medical teams control what you cannot and they can. Whoever or whatever controls your mind; will generally come out on top; your mental strength is the key to your outcome. Take care of yourself, take care of your mind, be strong, be resilient and be determined to see your recovery through to the end.

Note from the Author

Hi I'm a very experienced Personal Development Coach, Soft Skills Coach & Workplace Mental Health Well-being Practitioner. I believe that many concerns we have can be solved by how we approach them; and that ultimately starts with our mind set. Do you have a positive mind set or a negative mind set when you are faced with a situation that causes you stress?

The word stress can be used quite loosely, when someone's having a bad day or they have missed the bus to work- these feelings would generally be an inconvenience and an annoyance that would disappear as quickly as they came. In modern society we have come to find that life today is on average 44% more difficult than 30 years ago based on the number of significant life changes. We hear on a daily basis that stress is all around us, and stress is a sign of the times, but whilst some of us can cope with it or try to ignore it, many of us do not have time in our busy lives to notice the detrimental effects it can have on our health and well-being. People who suffer from Anxiety have proven that their pain threshold is lower than normal. This means they experience pain more easily than others which in turn will lead to stress. This has led to some startling statistics:

- About 75% of all time lost in the workplace is stress related.
- Up to 90% of all visits to primary care doctors are for stress related complaints.
- The NHS in the UK claim, anxiety and depression are the most common mental health problems, and the majority of cases are caused by stress. Research by mental health charities also suggests that a quarter of the population will have a mental health problem at some point in their lives.

As a coach I am willing to teach you what I know and accept that you are developing yourself to be the best you can be, to bringing about positive a change to your life. I understand what it is like just starting out on your journey and I work at your pace. I have a vast knowledge, not just from learning, from experience, understanding and real life situations; working in wide and varied scenarios; with each wanting the same outcome. A Positive Resolution to the situation they find themselves in, a positive mental well-being and reducing stress levels.

Everyone has dreams. Some people may be able to follow through with them and achieve what they want, while other people are often held back, due to internal fears, discouragement, criticism and low self-esteem. Life coaching helps you tap into your strengths and resources, in order to get what you want. It helps people discover their values and strengths and use these, in order to attain their goals. Thus, in turn, leads to greater happiness and fulfilment. A plan of action helps give you the necessary direction, momentum and motivation, in order to achieve your goals. Sometimes, goals may not be achieved. There are essentially two reasons for this: either the goal was unrealistic or your habits did not support the completion of the specified actions. Goals that are not backed up with a realistic action plan are never attained. In fact, even after tailoring an action plan to your needs, you may not have implemented the actions laid out in the plan. In the absence of a plan of action, goals remain dreams, without the accomplishments required, in order to turn these dreams into reality. Inconsistency, inner fears, limiting beliefs, a perceived lack of internal resources (for example, knowledge) and external resources (for example, money or time) often act as excuses for not completing actions.

Certifications & Qualifications

- Qualified & Accredited INLPTA Master Practitioner
- Qualified & Accredited SNLP Coach
- Qualified & Accredited Psychotherapist
- Qualified & Accredited Hypnotherapist
- Qualified & Accredited Life Coach

Contact me at leadingforsuccess@hotmail.com if you want to make those positive changes in your life.

Quote from a young lady who lost her mum to cancer three years ago, who read my book

"Had a read through, this message is amazing and really inspiring, some powerful lines really stand out and will resonate with so many people; just wanted you to let you know I think it's fab; your mentality is amazing. Maybe when you are feeling 100% you could look at combining some of your meditation/hypnosis experience with your own cancer experience and work with chemo patients to help them get mentally fit for their own cancer battles". Nu xxxx

Printed in Poland
by Amazon Fulfillment
Poland Sp. z o.o., Wrocław

53844740R00129